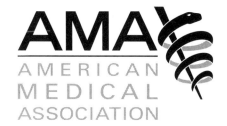

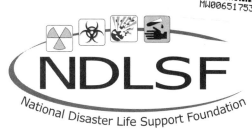

ADVANCED DISASTER LIFE SUPPORT™

v.3.0

Course Manual

Editor-in-Chief

John H. Armstrong, MD

Deputy Editor

Richard B. Schwartz, MD

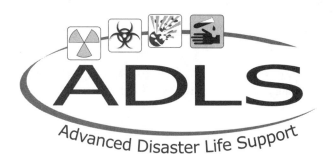

TABLE OF CONTENTS

CHAPTER | THREE

Health System Surge Capacity for Disasters and Public Health Emergencies

CHAPTER | FOUR

Community Health Emergency Operations and Response

CHAPTER | **FIVE**

Legal and Ethical Issues in Disasters

PREFACE

The increasing incidence of disasters around the globe reflects higher population density in disaster-prone areas, greater presence of hazardous materials in communities, emerging and continuing diseases, and enduring conflicts. Effective disaster preparation and response requires a disaster mindset, both individually and collectively, that recognizes the need for mass casualty and affected population management.

The Advanced Disaster Life Support™ (ADLS®) course version 3.0 continues the progression toward interprofessional disaster readiness through education and training of medical first responders, clinicians, public health professionals, and emergency managers. It builds on the combined framework of the PRE-DISASTER Paradigm™ and the DISASTER Paradigm™ from the Core Disaster Life Support® (CDLS®) course and the all-hazards clinical management of disaster casualties from the Basic Disaster life Support™ (BDLS®) course.

The ADLS v.3.0 course incorporates 28 disaster medicine and public health preparedness competencies as defined by Subbarao and colleagues in *Disaster Medicine and Public Health Preparedness* (2008). It applies National Disaster Life Support (NDLS) principles by moving beyond the care of the individual casualty to the management of the mass casualty population and the affected community. The ADLS v.3.0 course manual is an essential part of the course, and yet remains a useful resource beyond the course: it describes essential tools for effective disaster response, to include mass casualty and population-based triage, surge capacity and capability community health emergency operations, worker safety through personal protective equipment and decontamination, and algorithms for hazard-specific mass casualty care. The manual also provides the legal and ethical context for responsible disaster engagement.

The ADLS v.3.0 course provides standardized opportunities to practice each of the key tools for effective disaster response through table-top exercises, skills stations, and functional exercises. Successful course completion verifies cognitive performance and demonstration of disaster skills, and should stimulate ongoing preparedness activities: There is no finish line!

John H. Armstrong, MD
Editor-in-Chief, Advanced Disaster Life Support™ Version 3.0

Richard B. Schwartz, MD
Deputy Editor, Advanced Disaster Life Support™ Version 3.0

ACKNOWLEDGMENTS

The editors acknowledge the contributions toward the development of ADLS v.3.0 made by:

Scott Lillibridge, MD
Italo Subbarao, DO, MBA
Raymond E. Swienton, MD

The American Medical Association and the National Disaster Life Support Foundation, Inc., extend sincere appreciation to the founding authors and editors of the National Disaster Life Support course curricula for their continued vision and leadership in advancing and promoting excellence in education and training of all health care professionals in disaster medicine and public health preparedness:

Phillip L. Coule, MD
Cham E. Dallas, PhD
James J. James, MD, DrPH, MHA
Scott Lillibridge, MD
Paul E. Pepe, MD, MPH
Richard B. Schwartz, MD
Raymond E. Swienton, MD

Developed in collaboration with:

The National Disaster Life Support Education Consortium™
Medical College of Georgia
University of Texas, Southwestern Medical Center at Dallas
University of Texas, School of Public Health at Houston
University of Georgia

ABOUT THE EDITORS

About the Editor-in-Chief

John H. Armstrong, MD is Associate Professor of Surgery, Division of Acute Care Surgery, at the University of South Florida (USF); Surgical Director of the USF Health American College of Surgeons-Accredited Education Institute; and Medical Director of the USF Health Center for Advanced Medical Learning and Simulation (CAMLS). He has completed a Master Educator Fellowship and holds a faculty appointment at the Uniformed Services University of the Health Sciences.

Dr. Armstrong serves on the Executive Committee of the American Medical Association National Disaster Life Support Educational Consortium; is a founding editorial board member of the AMA journal, *Disaster Medicine and Public Health Preparedness*; and is a consultant to the American College of Surgeons (ACS) Ad Hoc Committee on Disaster Preparedness. He serves as Chair of the American College of Surgeons delegation to the AMA House of Delegates (HOD); ACS Governor from Florida; and member of the Accreditation Council for Graduate Medical Education Residency Review Committee for Surgery. He is a former trustee and executive committee member of the AMA.

About the Deputy Editor

Richard B. Schwartz, MD is Chairman and Professor of Emergency Medicine at Georgia Health Sciences University. Dr. Schwartz is one of the original creators of the National Disaster Life Support™ (NDLS™) series of courses and serves as the Vice Chairman of the National Disaster Life Support Foundation, Inc. He is board certified in Emergency Medicine and an accomplished educator, having developed national and international programs. He has considerable operational experience in the areas of Disaster and Tactical Medicine, and is well published in these areas. His research focus is in the fields of hemorrhage control, disaster triage, and airway management.

ABOUT THE CONTRIBUTORS

Dennis E. Amundson, DO, MS, practices Critical Care Medicine for Scripps Healthcare in San Diego. He is Board Certified and a Fellow in the American Board of Internal Medicine and has qualifications in Internal, Pulmonary and Critical Care Medicine. Captain (ret) Amundson was the first program director of a Critical Care Medicine Fellowship in the US Navy and served as a Surgeon General's Advisor for 10 years. Captain Amundson served as Pulmonary Department Head and Fellowship Director for the Navy's first combined Pulmonary/Critical Care Medicine Program at Naval Medical Center San Diego. Doctor Amundson has over 100 published articles, abstracts, and book chapters, and he remains actively involved in clinical research. He has a longstanding research interest in sepsis, acute lung injury, and new critical care technology.

Frederick M. Burkle, Jr., MD, MPH, DTM, is Senior Fellow and Scientist, the Harvard Humanitarian Initiative, Harvard School of Public Health and Senior Associate Faculty and Research Scientist, the Center for Refugee & Disaster Response, Johns Hopkins University Medical Institutes. He also served as a Senior Public Policy Scholar, Woodrow Wilson Center for International Scholars, Washington, DC (2008–2010).

Arthur Cooper, MD, MS is Professor of Surgery at the Columbia University College of Physicians & Surgeons, Director of Trauma & Pediatric Surgical Services at the Harlem Hospital Center, and Affiliate Faculty at the National Center for Disaster Preparedness of the Columbia University Mailman School of Public Health. He is a member of the Central Leadership Council of the New York City Pediatric Disaster Coalition, and a founding member of the American Board of Disaster Medicine, with expertise in the fields of pediatric trauma, disaster medicine, and emergency preparedness.

Edbert B. Hsu, MD, MPH is the Director of Training at the Johns Hopkins Office of Critical Event Preparedness and Response (CEPAR) and associate professor in the Department of Emergency Medicine. His research has focused on educational frameworks and hospital exercise evaluation.

Eric Robert Frykberg, MD is Professor of Surgery, University of Florida College of Medicine and Chief, Division of General Surgery at Shands Jacksonville Medical Center. Dr Frykberg served three years of active duty in the US Navy Medical Corps at Jacksonville Naval Hospital, after which he joined the faculty of the University of Florida College of Medicine at the Jacksonville campus in 1985, where he continues to serve as a core trauma surgeon. His major interests include vascular trauma and disaster management.

E. Brooke Lerner, PhD, is an injury epidemiologist and a former EMS field provider. She is currently an Associate Professor at the Medical College of Wisconsin in the Department of Emergency Medicine. She has nearly 20 years of EMS related experience and has authored dozens of EMS-related, peer-reviewed publications.

Jim Lyznicki, MS, MPH, is the associate director of the AMA Center for Public Health Preparedness and Disaster Response at the American Medical Association. He holds master's degrees in medical microbiology and in environmental and occupational health. Prior to the AMA, he spent 10 years as a clinical microbiology laboratory supervisor at the University of Chicago Medical Center and the Rush University Medical Center; and 2 years as an environmental health scientist at the University of Illinois School of Public Health.

Greene Shepherd, PhrmD is a clinical professor with Georgia's Health Science University. Dr. Shepherd is a diplomat of the American Board of Applied Toxicology and a Fellow of the American Academy of Clinical Toxicology. He has been involved with the NDLS program since 2003.

Frederick L. Slone, MD is the Medical Director for The Center for Advanced Clinical Learning at the University of South Florida (USF) College of Medicine and is responsible for simulation activities for USF. He has contributed to multiple published abstracts in the field of simulation. In addition, Dr. Slone is the Director for the National Disaster Life Support Foundation (NDLSF) Training Center at USF and is a Board Member of the American Board of Disaster Medicine.

Italo Subbarao, DO, MBA, is the Director of Public Health Readiness Office at the AMA Center for Public Health Preparedness and Disaster Response, Deputy Editor of *Disaster Medicine and Public Health Preparedness* journal, and Medical Director, National Disaster Life Support Program Office. Dr. Subbarao has expertise in health system recovery and promoting comprehensive disaster planning through private-public partnerships.

Meredith Hill Thanner, PhD is a Program Manager with Battelle Memorial Institute, Centers for Public Health Research and Evaluation. Dr. Thanner has experience in health system disaster preparedness and response and in sociological and public health research.

Matthew Wynia, MD, MPH, is an internist, a specialist in infectious diseases, and the Director of the Institute for Ethics at the American Medical Association. Dr. Wynia has done research, written and lectured extensively on public health and bioethics, including examining ethical issues in disaster response.

REVIEWERS

John H Clouse, MSR
University of Louisville School of Medicine

Arthur Cooper, MD, MS
Columbia University

Robert L. Ditch, Colonel, USAF, Ret, EdD (c), CEM, NREMT-P
Synaptic Emergency Educational Services &
The George Washington University

Alan Dobrowolski, RN
Regional Emergency Medical Services Authority/International Center for
Prehospital and Disaster Medicine

Arthur J. French, MD, Captain, U.S. Public Health Service (Ret.)
Veterans Health Administration

Chu Hyun Kim, MD
Inje University College of Medicine

Thomas D Kirsch, MD, MPH
Johns Hopkins University

Craig Llewellyn, MD, MDTM & H
Uniformed Services University of Health Sciences School of Medicine

Lewis W Marshall Jr., MS, MD, JD, LLM
Brookdale University Medical Center

Michael McLaughlin, PhD, NREMT-P
Kirkwood College

Consuelo M. Maxim, BSHSA, EMT-P
Muskegon County Medical Control Authority

David Nitsch, BS, NREMT-P
Albert Einstein Medical Center

Kevin O'Hara, MS, EMT-P
Nassau County EMS Academy and
Stony Brook University Medical Center

James Paturas, CEM, EMT-P, CBCP
Yale New Haven Center for Emergency Preparedness and Disaster Response

Steven J Parrillo, DO
Philadelphia University
Albert Einstein Healthcare Network

Deborah J Persell, PhD, RN, APN
Arkansas State University Regional Training Center for
Disaster Preparedness Education

Stephen Phillipe Sr., BS, LEM
Louisiana Department of Health, Bureau of EMS

Heather Seemann, NREMT-P, FP-C, CCP-C, MLT(ASCP)
North Slope Borough Fire Department

Lee B Smith, MD, JD
West Virginia University

Andrew E. Spain, MA, NCEE, CCP-C
University of Missouri

Ricardo Tappan, CSHM, FF/NREMT
George Washington Medical Faculty Associates

COURSE OBJECTIVES

Upon completion of the Advanced Disaster Life Support™ (ADLS™) course, participants will be able to:

➤ Explain the shift from individual-to population-based care in a disaster or public health emergency. *(Chapter 1)*

➤ Practice mass casualty triage in a simulated disaster scenario. *(Chapter 2)*

➤ Choose strategies to establish organizational and community surge capacity in a disaster or public health emergency. *(Chapter 3)*

➤ Differentiate roles performed in an emergency operations center or incident command center established in response to a simulated mass casualty event. *(Chapter 4)*

➤ Discuss legal, regulatory, and ethical principles and practices to enable health professionals to provide crisis standards of care in a disaster or public health emergency. *(Chapter 5)*

➤ Select personal protective equipment and decontamination measures appropriate for personnel and public health protection in a disaster or public health emergency. *(Chapter 6)*

➤ Apply clinical skills for the management of mass casualties in simulated all-hazards scenarios. *(Chapter 7)*

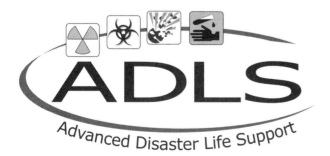

CHAPTER | ONE

Disasters and Public Health Emergencies

Edbert B. Hsu, MD, MPH

Jim Lyznicki, MS, MPH

Italo Subbarao, DO, MBA

Meredith Thanner, PhD

Frederick M. Burkle, Jr., MD, MPH, DTM

1.1 PURPOSE

Large-scale disasters and public health emergencies shift the focus from individual- to population-based care or, put another way, from individual patients to mass casualties. This chapter emphasizes the public health consequences of disasters and reviews the DISASTER Paradigm™ as a common framework for addressing mass casualty and population-based care across the clinical, public health, and emergency response sectors.

1.2 LEARNING OBJECTIVES

After completing this chapter, readers will be able to:

➤ Discuss the rationale for including public health emergencies as essential operational elements of modern disaster classification.

➤ Explain the need to evaluate, describe, and monitor the public health impact of disasters, specifically on measurable direct and indirect mortality and morbidity.

➤ Discuss the elements of the DISASTER Paradigm in the context of providing mass casualty and population-based care.

1.3   DISASTER MEDICINE AND PUBLIC HEALTH PREPAREDNESS COMPETENCY ADDRESSED[1]

➤ Describe the all-hazards framework for disaster planning and mitigation. (1.1.1)

1.4   INTRODUCTION

The effects of disasters and public health emergencies can be studied empirically through well-established clinical and epidemiologic research methods. Such information is critical for the development of clinical and public health preparedness, response, and recovery plans. Evidence should inform the discipline of disaster medicine and public health preparedness, and ongoing research is needed to elucidate the clinical and public health effects of specific disasters; analyze risk factors for adverse social and health effects; and assess the effectiveness of clinical and public health interventions, disaster assistance, and relief operations on the long-term restoration or improvement of predisaster conditions.

In the early 1970s, published literature on disasters was largely anecdotal and descriptive with a dearth of peer-reviewed, scientific research on the causes and management of disasters. In the decade that followed, many research studies began to appear, beginning a plethora of investigations that have rapidly advanced the expanding discipline of disaster medicine and public health preparedness beyond expectations. The 1980s and 1990s saw the proliferation of disaster journals, professional associations, funded research agendas, and interests of governments in mitigating disaster impacts. Today, thousands of peer-reviewed studies have been published worldwide in more than 700 different journals that include medicine, public health, nursing, prehospital care, mental health, social sciences, and emergency management.

Initially, studies focused on mastering the response to, and management of, disasters by increasing skill sets for a professional base of responders. Most developed countries have basic competence and experience in disaster management, yet they face large gaps in mitigation and preparedness. The least developed countries have the greatest prevalence of lethal disasters due to high-risk geography, poverty, limited infrastructure, and ineffective government. As such, many countries have progressed little in their capacity to limit the morbidity (injury and illness) and mortality (deaths) of their populations in disasters; too frequently, the only experienced aid is international. Much remains to be done in predisaster education, training, prevention, and planning, as well as in operationally recognizing the importance of disaster medicine and public health preparedness as a discipline in support of global health.

1.5 THE EVOLVING NATURE OF DISASTERS AND PUBLIC HEALTH EMERGENCIES

Disaster impacts, most commonly measured as "direct consequences" related to the impact of the disaster itself, include mortality, morbidity, and psychological stress. Violations of international law protections are also direct consequences, especially in conflict-related disasters in the least developed countries with disenfranchised and vulnerable minorities.

In the early years of disaster management, emphasis was placed on developing skills to reduce direct consequences. Since then, disaster professionals have gained a better understanding of the public health and social science consequences of disasters. These consequences are "indirect" and reflect the breakdown of health care and social services, systems, and infrastructure. Loss of the most essential elements of life, including food, water, shelter, and clothing, may lead to increased population mortality and morbidity. Indirect consequences are rarely the subject of disaster planning or political attention and, for the most part, remain undetected, unmeasured, and unevaluated.

Fundamentally, public health emergencies can be defined as events that adversely impact the public health system and/or its protective infrastructure (ie, water, sanitation, shelter, food, fuel, and health), resulting in both direct and indirect consequences to the health of a population.[2,3] In the affected population, there is a high probability of a large number of deaths, a high number of serious or long-term disabled people, and wide exposure of a sizeable number of people at risk for future harm. The focus in a public health emergency should be on promoting the capabilities of health systems, communities, and individuals to prevent, protect against, respond to, and recover from the event, particularly as the scale, timing, and unpredictability threaten to overwhelm routine capabilities.[4] From the moment that a disaster is recognized, both the acute medical care and public health systems need to be engaged for response.

Operationally, timely and accurate recognition of the public health impact is critical for prevention, preparedness, planning, and response. Certainly, not all disasters qualify as public health emergencies. "Potential injury- and/or illness-creating events" (PICE) are those that may initially appear to be static, well-controlled local events and yet may quickly become regional, national, or global disasters of paralytic proportions.[5,6] The PICE nomenclature provides a method for consistency in disaster classification, based on the potential for casualties, the impact on local medical capabilities, and the extent of geographic involvement. Severity, as indicated by rising disaster-fatality rates, increases as resources become limited and disaster discriminators (eg, widespread geography, large affected population, prolonged timeline) push the emergence of a public health emergency (Table 1-1). Identical disasters may have differing consequences depending on the location of the event and the availability of resources. Circumstances that may first result in direct injuries and death may change rapidly, causing excess indirect illness and subsequent death as essential public health resources deteriorate, are destroyed, or are systematically denied to vulnerable populations. Consequences often impact entire communities, and, thus, solutions must be population-based. In most events, indirect consequences are preventable. Ultimately, indirect mortality and morbidity may be the most sensitive indicators of quality performance in disaster planning and response efforts.

Factors that move a disaster event toward becoming a public health emergency with exacerbation of injuries and/or illnesses include[7]:

➤ Widespread geography.

➤ Large population size and density.

➤ Prolonged time with exposure to the disaster.

➤ Deficient or absent preexisting public health infrastructure to respond to crises.

➤ Compromised public health capacity and capability as a result of the disaster.

➤ Existing ecological and environmental decay.

➤ Adverse environment created by the disaster.

TABLE 1-1 Range of Disasters and Public Health Emergencies Based on Time, Scale, and Health Outcomes

DISASTERS*		
Event characteristics	**Potential injury-creating events**	**Potential illness-creating events**
➤ Deliberate or unintentional ➤ Geographically limited ➤ Population limited ➤ Time limited	Direct and indirect morbidity and mortality from: ➤ Bombings and explosions ➤ Weather-related natural disasters ➤ Geophysical natural disasters	Direct and indirect morbidity and mortality from: ➤ Isolated bioevents (outbreaks) ➤ Chemical and radiologic events

*These events may never be totally prevented. However, both direct and indirect consequences of injury- and illness- (including mental health and psychosocial) creating events can be kept at a minimum without resulting in a public health emergency through good planning, prevention, and response. For example, the current Global Public Health Information Network (GPHIN) provides daily early warning of worldwide outbreaks, successfully preventing most from reaching epidemic status.

PUBLIC HEALTH EMERGENCIES**		
Event characteristics	**Potential injury-creating events**	**Potential illness-creating events**
➤ Deliberate or unintentional ➤ Geographically widespread	Direct and indirect morbidity and mortality from: ➤ War and conflict	Direct and indirect morbidity and mortality from: ➤ Epidemics/pandemics

	PUBLIC HEALTH EMERGENCIES**	
Event characteristics	Potential injury-creating events	Potential illness-creating events
➤ Large population affected ➤ Prolonged duration	➤ Nuclear weapon detonation ➤ Large-scale radiologic/ chemical disasters ➤ Large-scale natural disasters ➤ Weather-related ➤ Geophysical	➤ Climate change-related events ➤ Drought and famine ➤ Secondary consequence of injury-creating events

**These event discriminators allow for a public health emergency to occur either directly (eg, as a consequence of a pandemic or famine) or indirectly (eg, as a consequence of destroyed, inadequate, or denied public health protections: infrastructure or systems). Characteristically, indirect consequences (eg, preventable illnesses, disabilities, mental and psychosocial illness) exceed direct causes and persist for many years after the precipitating event.

Source: Adapted from Burkle and Greenough[7]

1.6 DISASTER TAXONOMY: REVIEW OF DISASTERS AND PUBLIC HEALTH EMERGENCIES

Taxonomy in disaster classification describes distinguishing characteristics, as well as common relationships, among disasters. While a number of disaster classifications exist, the most inclusive taxonomy defines three distinct categories: natural disasters, human systems (technological) failures, and conflict-based disasters (Table 1-2).

Some disasters straddle multiple categories (ie, natural disasters and human systems failures).[7] Hurricane Katrina (2005) was a natural disaster, yet the failure of the levees with flooding and subsequent infrastructure loss was a human systems failure. The combination of the two produced an unprecedented public health emergency.

By compartmentalizing disasters into current taxonomies, disaster planners may fail to recognize complex, multidimensional elements and, as a consequence, miss direct and indirect effects. The distinction between natural and technological disasters can become blurred, as in the case of industrial catastrophes, structural collapse of buildings, transportation-related emergencies, release of hazardous materials by fires or explosions, and infectious disease outbreaks. Dealing with these commonly occurring events requires an all-hazards approach to disaster prevention and management to coordinate better planning and effective response.

1.6.1 Natural (Geophysical) Disasters

Natural disasters result from natural forces and represent the prototype of injury-creating events. They are referred to as "incidents" or "local disasters"

TABLE 1-2 Disaster Categories

Disaster Category	Examples
Natural (Geophysical)	➤ Earthquake ➤ Hurricane ➤ Blizzards & ice storms ➤ Landslide ➤ Tornado ➤ Volcano ➤ Natural outbreak of infectious disease
Human Systems Failure (Technological)	➤ Airplane crash ➤ Chemical release or spill ➤ Nuclear plant meltdown ➤ Train derailment ➤ Building collapse
Conflict	➤ Civil disturbance ➤ Complex emergency ➤ Terrorism (including bioterrorism) ➤ War

in that their impact is immediate and direct, while the time course, population, and geography are limited. The direct medical consequence is the mass casualty incident (MCI) or mass casualty event (MCE); in the former, the casualty load strains resources, while in the latter, resources are clearly overwhelmed by the casualties. Hundreds of MCIs occur annually, and most are characterized by direct traumatic injuries, with the majority of casualties not being critically injured. Casualties receive care in existing local or regional facilities or, less commonly, supplemental services from outside humanitarian agencies and organizations.

Most natural disasters are similar in that they are limited in scale and time, and managed locally with subsequent infusion of regional or national resources as needed. In the developed world, natural disasters rarely result in a public health emergency unless they affect the public health infrastructure and system (eg, Indian Ocean tsunami, 2004; Hurricane Katrina in the Gulf of Mexico, 2005; and Haiti earthquake, 2010). Large-scale natural disasters have the potential to cause considerable direct and indirect mortality, particularly in rapidly growing, dense urban populations living in the disaster-prone zones (coastal, lowland, active fault, volcanic) of Asia, Africa, and the Americas.

Public health emergencies following natural disasters are more commonly encountered in developing countries, in which essential public health and health care services are already deficient or absent at baseline. This includes overcrowding of camps and shelters for displaced populations, insufficient sanitary facilities, and flooding, all of which can stress water supplies and enable illnesses, such as the 2010 cholera outbreak in post-earthquake Haiti. Natural disasters that become public health emergencies are likely to be geographically widespread and prolonged, and often occur where population densities have increased without infrastructure accommodation or improvement. Such antecedent ecological and environmental instability limits the ability of the ecosystem to absorb the shock.

Natural disasters frequently alter the macrobiotic and microbiotic environments, either introducing new disease pathogens or increasing the opportunity for existing pathogens to infect humans. As an example, the landslides and aftershocks generated from the Northridge, California, earthquake (1994) created dust clouds that led to an increased incidence of endemic coccidioidomycosis infections.

Epidemics and pandemics are always public health emergencies. They are characterized by large numbers of people seeking health care. The population thus becomes the focus of management in this situation. Effective management under these circumstances requires a shift in mindset away from the individual patient and toward the affected population. Such a shift does not minimize the importance of clinical care but rather adds the dimension of public health and surge-capacity interventions that improve population *access* to *available* limited health resources. All individuals within a population share the following circumstances[12]:

➤ All have the same condition or are susceptible to it.

➤ All have shared health care needs.

➤ All require some intervention ranging from preventive education to critical care.

➤ All fall into one of five triage-management categories: *s*usceptible, *e*xposed, *i*nfectious, *r*emoved by death or illness recovery, or *v*accine protected (SEIRV).

Large-scale pandemics may require a sustained operational response lasting 12 to 24 months. Pandemics readily elude a compromised health information and surveillance system, and rapidly stress already overwhelmed or poorly resourced public health infrastructures and systems. Before the events of September 11, 2001, few US health departments had adequate outbreak investigation and control resources or surveillance systems that were sensitive to emerging and reemerging diseases. Lessons from the outbreak of severe acute respiratory syndrome in 2003 and the H1N1 influenza pandemic in 2009–2010 demonstrated the need for close integration of medical and public health authorities to ensure a functioning global surveillance system, crucial for identifying and tracking disease outbreaks and assisting countries in disease prevention and control. It is important to recognize that a pandemic refers only to the distribution of the disease; the degree to which a pandemic presents a public health emergency is also related to its transmissibility, its severity, and the population's susceptibility.

Natural Disasters: Progress or Peril

➤ In the 2010 Port au Prince Haiti, earthquake, dense populations living on the deforested hillsides were more prone to direct consequences (death and injury) than those who lived elsewhere. Only 1% of Haiti's surface cover includes protective tree roots, so the environment is intolerant of heavy rains as well—mudslides and severe flooding with drowning are common consequences.

➤ The 2004 Indian Ocean tsunami affected 20 countries. More than five years later, many countries lack recovery and rehabilitation of essential health services and facilities, potable water, shelter, and health care workers. Indirect mortality and morbidity are inevitable consequences.

➤ More than 70 new or reemerging infectious diseases have occurred this past decade. Population density and ease of travel allow for the rapid transmission of pathogens. Public health surveillance systems are critical for monitoring existing and emerging disease outbreaks. Few developing countries have adequate surveillance systems, and those in the United States that were bolstered after the terrorist attacks in fall 2001 have deteriorated from recent lack of funding.

1.6.2   Human Systems (Technological) Failures

These disasters result from significant human failure in any portion of a system, including input (eg, human design failure), process (eg, material failure), and output (eg, release of toxic fumes), and they cause physical destruction, direct mortality and morbidity, population displacement, and environmental contamination. In developed countries, successful management of human-caused biologic, chemical, radiation, and explosive events is dependent on an adequate surveillance system and response capability. To date, most of these incidents have been handled well by local, regional, and national authorities, with some events requiring acute international and technically-specialized agency assistance.

Because of inadequate systems for outbreak investigation, surveillance, and control capacities, infectious disease outbreaks risk becoming epidemics in developing countries. Combined national assets in partnership with World Health Organization–fielded emergency response teams have contained H5N1 and H1N1 influenza outbreaks, but the risk of spread continues globally, especially in countries where culture, poverty, and politics clash with limited and fragile public health protection. Too often, international assistance from advantaged countries is ad hoc, inconsistent, and politically motivated, all of which represent failures in human systems.

Barring unusual circumstances, similar response capacity is expected in developed countries where chemical and radiation disasters occur. The 1986 Chernobyl nuclear plant explosion was a unique human systems failure disaster resulting from a flawed reactor design, compromised response with inadequately trained personnel, and disregard for personnel safety. Five percent of the radioactive reactor core was released into the atmosphere; there were 47 direct deaths from radiation and thermal burns and nine indirect deaths from thyroid cancer. Twenty years after the disaster, two United Nations (UN) reports (2000; 2005–2006) concluded that the public health effects were not as substantial as had first been feared. Yet another estimate of long-term indirect deaths, approaching 4000, demonstrates that indirect deaths remain untracked and unnoticed. In the 1984 Bhopal, India, industrial disaster, 3000 direct deaths occurred immediately, with 15,000 to 20,000 indirect deaths occurring over the next two decades. As underscored by the 1987 Goiania, Brazil, cesium 137 radiation incident, other consequences across psychosocial, economic, and legal domains must be monitored as well.

Human systems failures in public health infrastructure and processes greatly contribute to the indirect effects of natural disasters. In the latter part of the 20th century, natural disasters from prolonged drought in Africa and Asia catalyzed famines, which were subsequently exacerbated by war, misguided internal economic policies, and external political exigencies. Examples include Cambodia in the 1970s, Ethiopia in the 1980s, and North Korea in the 1990s. The unheeded levee structure warnings before Hurricane Katrina, and the lack of tsunami-sensing and early-warning devices in underwater earthquake-prone areas, illustrate human systems failures to take preventive action. Although globalization has led to economic improvements in the developing world, it has also led to greater gaps in health, education, and wealth among the "have" and "have not" populations in the same countries. These effects are often not demonstrated until inequities in predisaster protections and postdisaster health care are exposed.

Cyclone Nargis (2009) typifies a human systems failure "perfect storm": the expansive delta area of Myanmar that had been deforested of its protective mangrove forests in favor of shrimp farms and rice paddies; a warming Indian Ocean that enabled a surge 25 miles inland due to raging storm intensity, heavier rainfall, and low vertical wind shear; an impoverished population densely clustered along the delta; and a government that had not invested in essential public health, leading to chronic malnutrition in 31% to 61% across the population.

Human Systems (Technological) Failures: Progress or Peril

➤ While the origins of climate change continue to be debated, Polynesian islands are disappearing because of a rise in sea level and the acidification collapse of their reef ecosystems. Rainwater storage wells, lagoons, and coastal areas are contaminated and polluted with elevated bacterial counts, resulting in central urbanization and mounting economic and food challenges. The island nation of Kiribati, which straddles the equator, is being slowly evacuated. By 2050, it is expected that 75 million islanders will migrate.[13]

➤ There are 34 biodiversity areas of the world that are home to sensitive plants and vertebrates necessary for the earth's agricultural and food sustainability. Eighty percent of recent wars have occurred in 23 of these biodiversity hotspots, and few of these spots have recovered.[13]

➤ Megacities modify their own ecosystems. Rapid urbanization with replacement of soil by asphalt and concrete causes "heat islands" that absorb sunlight. For each percentage point of urban growth, there is a 2.44 mm decrease in rainfall. Rainfall that does occur is not absorbed into the land, and runoff contributes to floods and contamination.[13]

➤ In April 2010, an explosion on the British Petroleum–leased Deepwater Horizon oil rig killed 11 workers and left several others injured. Yet the magnitude of this technological failure only grew when the rig sank within 2 days of the explosion and oil from the well began spilling toward the Gulf Coast. The extent of the oil spill is unprecedented, and the human and environmental health impacts in the affected region remain unknown. It is recognized, however, that the environmental effects from the Exxon Valdez oil tanker spill in Prince William Sound, Alaska, in March 1989 linger 20 years later.[14]

1.6.3   Conflict-Based Disasters

Conflict-based disasters and human systems failures are separated only by intent. A conflict-based disaster involves the intentional creation of human insecurity by actual or threatened terrorism, civil disorder along political, ethnic, religious, or economic lines, or war with large-scale loss of life. The 2005 United Nations (UN) World Summit authorized the international community to protect vulnerable populations from these disasters through the collective action of the UN Security Council, but the reality is that nation-state sovereignty rights remain unclear, leading to inaction, delayed action, or inadequate intervention to safeguard affected peoples.[13]

War is the prototype for the study of public health emergencies. Direct deaths from war-related violence rarely exceed 10% (range, <2% to 29%) of the total mortality; indirect health consequences predominate due to population displacement, disrupted food supplies and food security, destroyed health facilities and public health infrastructure, and ruined livelihoods. The resultant indirect mortality rates are rarely measured and receive little political attention. Most direct mortality in war zones occurs where eyewitnesses are least likely to go. The media are often the only source of data and are able to gather 30% of all direct deaths through research of mass graves, missing persons, and Ministry of Health morgue and health facility reports. In extremely violent wars, media reports may not pick up more than 5% of the direct deaths.[13]

Internal wars are politically motivated disasters that result in high levels of violence, civilian deaths, "ethnic cleansing" and genocide, and public health catastrophes. They dominated the last third of the 20th century, when more people were killed by forces from within their own country than from outside. Genocidal and ethnic cleansing deaths were primarily from direct violence in Rwanda, Cambodia, Sudan, Bosnia, and Kosovo. In other conflicts with less direct violence, such as the former Yugoslavia, Iraq, Gaza, and the Democratic Republic of Congo, religious and ethnic minorities were consistently denied basic protections in food, water, shelter, and health; the result was an increasing pattern of indirect mortality and morbidity. Conflicts that led to refugee migrations or internally displaced populations resulted in deaths related to poor public health (eg, cholera and dysentery among Rwandan refugees in the former Zaire). Among civilians, indirect deaths from war-exacerbated malnutrition and disease exceeded violent deaths by a sizeable margin.[13]

Combat deaths drive outside political and humanitarian interventions. As mortality declines, so does outside interest and relief aid. After the shooting stops, direct deaths decline rapidly, yet indirect mortality and morbidity continue to increase from lack of access to, and availability of, health care and other essential services. These may not return to baseline for more than a decade. Suicide, depression, alcohol and drug abuse, and gender-based violence are common markers of ongoing community breakdown and economic and physical insecurity. Premature childhood deaths, especially among girls, occur when families are unable to afford education and health protection; preventable infectious diseases, such as human immunodeficiency virus, tuberculosis, and malaria, often reemerge or worsen due to government and economic failures. Dengue outbreaks can occur from inadequate trash removal tied to postconflict-induced urban decay. In prolonged wars, women and children are the most common long-term casualties.[13]

While the number of direct and indirect deaths from declared internal wars has declined markedly in this century, the number of serious hotspots within the developing and developed world remains high. Deaths from slowly escalating political violence and state repression, diminished access to health care, and degraded public health protections in these internal hotspots will likely remain unnoticed unless the conflict widens or mass population displacements occur. Civil wars during the past 40 years have not brought positive social change, but have left legacies of high economic and social costs, borne by civilians and compounded long after the wars are over (eg, Sierra Leone, Liberia, Angola, Uganda, and Cambodia). The primary objective of insurgents in civil war is to control a population, not necessarily territory or resources.

Another contributor to indirect morbidity and mortality in conflict-based and natural disasters in developing countries is the pervasive lack of food to sustain basic health—that level of macronutrition and micronutrition necessary for homeostasis. For the more than 1 billion people who are food insecure, food assistance often does not reach their affected regions early enough to avert widespread hunger; the food that does arrive may not yield full rations or may be culturally unfamiliar or unacceptable. Humanitarian assistance has also moved increasingly to urban enclaves as African and Asian populations seek health, safety, and security by moving from rural to urban areas. Thus, rural food assistance is severely limited, and these areas become extremely vulnerable to indirect consequences of disasters.

Terrorism generates direct health effects when used in isolation or in asymmetric warfare. Examples include suicide bombers in Pakistan and Israel, where a population mass is targeted, or combatants detonating roadside devices in Iraq and Afghanistan. However, such explosions themselves and other mechanisms of terror (biologic, chemical, and radiologic) generate indirect effects, ranging from delayed and protracted illness to severe and protracted mental health consequences. "Dirty bombs" combine a nonnuclear explosive with radioactive material and are intended to create local injury and widespread panic.

Nuclear blasts include low- and high-yield nuclear explosions, the latter having the potential to generate tens of thousands of casualties for whom the limited medical resources will have little effect. Casualty numbers in high-yield nuclear blasts will greatly exceed surviving medical resources; an expectation of one surviving physician for every 400 to 900 casualties might be high. Organized life-saving operations and essential public health and agricultural infrastructure will not be available. The Cold War goal of preselected triage criteria was to identify the more certain "survival possible" casualties from among the living: those with minor injuries (expected to live without intervention) would be included, and those with acute radiation exposure (and expected to die) would be excluded. Long-term triage was designed to save a culture, the recoverable public health and agricultural infrastructure, and government structures in order to mitigate indirect mortality and morbidity.

Conflict-Based Disasters: Progress or Peril

➤ All wars of the last three decades have resulted in more deaths from destroyed public health infrastructure protections and preventable diseases than from the direct impact of weaponry. Both Iraq and Afghanistan illustrate the pervasive insecurity from asymmetric warfare that prevents effective and efficient humanitarian aid from being delivered. In Iraq, indirect deaths began to grow as the public health catastrophe penetrated the fragile Iraqi society, yet remained below the threshold of public awareness. In less than five years, Iraq, considered to have had a developed national health system, sustained declining health indices consistent with those found in the most undeveloped countries. Afghanistan's both direct and indirect mortality and morbidity rates will never be accurately measured, but with half the country remaining insecure and without benefit of outside aid, a public health catastrophe continues to unfold.

➤ Today, more internally displaced populations exist than ever in the history of the world. Populations fleeing lingering conflict, postwar poverty, and environmental change have rapidly populated African and Asian cities. This rapid urbanization is unsustainable because the population increase has outstripped available public health protections. Sanitation is ignored, and infectious diseases become more prevalent. The highest infant and early childhood mortality rates are now found in urban settings.

1.6.4 Combined Disasters

While conceptualizing disasters across natural, technological, and conflict categories is a useful construct, some catastrophic events are characterized by a combination of disasters from different categories and/or within the same category. Recent examples include Haiti in 2010 (natural disaster of an earthquake followed by an outbreak of cholera); and Japan in 2011 (natural disasters of earthquake and tsunami coupled with technological failure of radioactive leaks from nuclear reactors). These multiple mechanisms of disaster generate exponentially increased population needs and magnify the complexity of effective response.

1.7 NEED FOR A COMMON FRAMEWORK FOR MANAGEMENT OF DISASTERS AND PUBLIC HEALTH EMERGENCIES

The concept of public health emergencies is an essential operational element of modern disaster classification. Indirect morbidity and mortality is rarely the subject of planning and political attention; this underscores the notion that taxonomists, planners, and managers have not fully recognized the critical importance of indirect consequences in decision making. Many who call themselves disaster professionals have not experienced a public health emergency or participated in disaster operations at any level. In part, this is because most mass casualty incidents in both developed and developing countries are managed locally and regionally and do not progress to public health emergencies.

With an increase in global risk, clinical and public health professionals in all countries must be prepared for disasters and public health emergencies. The National Disaster Life Support™ (NDLS™) program recognizes the importance of **p**lanning and practice, **r**esilience, and **e**ducation and training (the PRE-DISASTER Paradigm™) across clinical and public health paradigms as a way to set conditions for success in disaster response and recovery (the DISASTER Paradigm).

Advanced disaster education and training emphasizes the elements of mitigation, preparation, response, and recovery in the management of public health crises, and directs attention to the direct and indirect health effects resulting from natural disasters, human systems failures, or conflict-based disasters. Formally recognizing health consequences in disaster taxonomy enables better planning and management of disasters. The Advanced Disaster Life Support (ADLS) course addresses disaster management and casualty care through a lens that brings focus to mass casualty *and* population-based health requirements.

Hurricane Katrina along the US Gulf Coast was a mass casualty disaster from wind and flooding, and a large-scale public health emergency from the acute loss of an already inadequate health care system. A key lesson from the response was the need for an interoperable and integrated health system to mitigate direct and indirect mortality and morbidity. Such a system works through a framework that enables clinical professionals, the public health workforce, emergency management services, and other response personnel to work as coordinated partners for effective disaster preparedness and response.

1.8 THE DISASTER PARADIGM™, MASS CASUALTY MANAGEMENT, AND POPULATION-BASED RESPONSE

The US public and private health sectors have considerable resources that can be used to help individuals and communities prepare for, respond to, and recover from disasters and public health emergencies. Following the terrorist attacks on September 11, 2001, the United States intensified efforts to improve the systems responsible for protecting and ensuring the health, safety, and well-being of individuals and communities in a disaster. Countless programs were developed to better resource, educate, and train health responders for terrorism and other mass casualty events.

Then, in 2005, Hurricane Katrina hit. Along with the human anguish and socio-economic damage left behind, illusions about the ability to launch a systematic, integrated health response were shattered. In the aftermath of the hurricane, various health-related issues surfaced at a magnitude not previously experienced by local and state health officials. Traditional response and recovery operations could not meet all of the resulting human needs, in either the short or long term. Addressing the diversity of "acute on chronic" health concerns, language and cultural barriers, and socioeconomic circumstances presented multiple challenges for disaster response and recovery systems.

Once a disaster occurs, the response phase involves implementation of personal, facility, and community disaster plans. Facility and community response plans should be implemented through a defined incident management structure, which may scale according to the disaster situation. Federal, state, and local government agencies have unmatched resources and legal authority to address disaster-related needs. Governments' authorities can coordinate extensive logistical efforts, such as moving large amounts of relief supplies. The NDLS program promotes a useful mnemonic, the DISASTER Paradigm, to identify the key elements of disaster response and recovery (Figure 1-1).

Application of the DISASTER Paradigm assists professionals from the clinical care, public health, and emergency management fields in responding to disaster with a structured, unifying approach across settings. This preestablished alignment facilitates the recognition and management of a mass casualty event and promotes the goal of providing the greatest good for the greatest number of casualties. The paradigm emphasizes an all-hazards approach to responding to a mass casualty event and facilitates a real-time and ongoing assessment of the incident scene. Advanced Disaster Life Support extends the use of the DISASTER Paradigm beyond the scene; thus, a review of the DISASTER Paradigm is appropriate.

1.8.1   Detection

The DISASTER Paradigm begins with *detection* of an incident. The detection stage requires situational awareness, including information management and communication, from both a clinical and a community perspective. This is vital

FIGURE 1-1

The DISASTER Paradigm

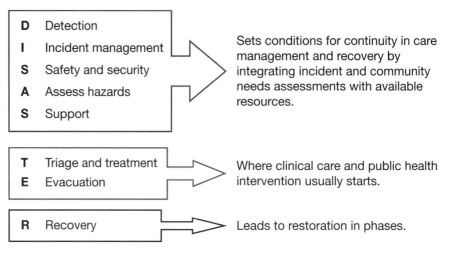

D Detection	Sets conditions for continuity in care management and recovery by integrating incident and community needs assessments with available resources.
I Incident management	
S Safety and security	
A Assess hazards	
S Support	
T Triage and treatment	Where clinical care and public health intervention usually starts.
E Evacuation	
R Recovery	Leads to restoration in phases.

Courtesy John H. Armstrong, MD, FACS.

for establishing a coordinated plan to respond to, as well as prevent expansion of, a mass casualty disaster.[15] This type of activity can be part of a broader ongoing monitoring program (eg, through emergency department screening, integration of hospital electronic medical records, and environmental biosensors) or can be conducted when an incident occurs by using rapid needs assessment tools that analyze the epidemiologic characteristics of casualties and define critical public health needs.

Other needs to be assessed include public access to shelter, water, sanitation, and health care, and the extent of damage to health care facilities. Though these tools should yield information regarding casualty needs, they should also be understandable and usable by nonmedical personnel. Whatever tools are used for detection, it is essential that they (1) have high specificity (low false–positive rate) and sensitivity (low false–negative rate) and (2) be able to capture and correlate data elements in a timely manner.[16] As these assessments are conducted, a safe distance from the disaster site must be maintained until the source of the incident is identified, and first responders are prepared to enter the area donning appropriate protective gear. The final element of the detection stage involves alerting authorities within the existing response system about the occurrence of an event and its cause. Many field technologies using voice, video, and data communication devices are available for such purposes.[16]

1.8.2   Incident Management

Once an incident has been detected and communicated to first-line responders, the next step in the DISASTER Paradigm is the establishment of an *incident management* structure. Incident management applies the principles of the incident command system (ICS) to establish an orderly chain of command with clearly defined roles, functions, and lines of communication to coordinate response and recovery efforts during most disasters; the more traditional ICS, however, may require further adaptation for management of a large-scale, prolonged health-related disaster, such as a pandemic.[16] The operational template for the effective management of an incident is the National Incident Management System (NIMS), which links responders and Emergency Operations Center (EOC) personnel from multiple jurisdictions (local, state, and federal) to facilitate coordinated response based on common information (Figure 1-2). Community emergency operations are described in more detail in Chapter 4.

Use of an ICS as a management tool for structuring the activity of disaster response agencies minimizes confusion by centralizing the processes of planning, operations, logistics, and finance. With an ICS, multiple and varied organizations are brought together under one clear management structure. This allows for the effective administration of diverse resources as needed across a complex and volatile emergency situation.[17] A number of evaluations of the ICS have recently been conducted; Buck and colleagues found that ICS "works best when those utilizing it are part of a community, when the demands being responded to are routine to them, and when social and cultural emergence is at a minimum. The ICS does not create a universally applicable bureaucratic organization among responders but rather is a mechanism for inter-organizational

FIGURE 1-2
Incident Management[16]

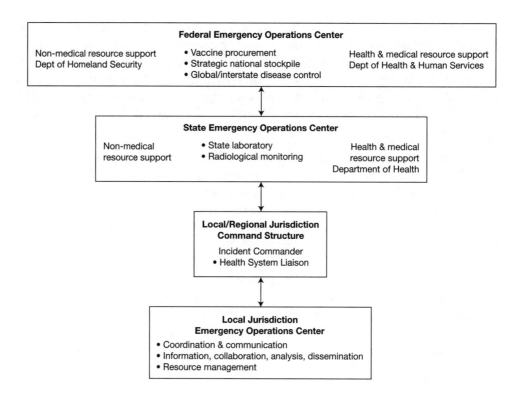

coordination designed to impose order on certain dimensions of the chaotic organizational environments of disasters."[18]

1.8.3   Safety and Security

As previously described, securing the incident scene is critical to ensuring the safety of those in the immediate area, including bystanders as well as first responders. Being able to identify *safety and security* threats, in the context of the event, allows for a faster and more effective initiation of response.[19] It is essential that responders keep their own safety, as well as that of their team members, as the top priority; rescue and health care operations can become severely compromised if first responders and health care workers become injured themselves. Injured responders become casualties with resource needs and reduce response resources at the same time.[20]

Responders must approach the scene with adequate protection before attempting to protect other groups, including the uninjured public and casualties. Responders can protect themselves by utilizing personal protective equipment (PPE), performing medical decontamination, and maintaining environmental vigilance. Part of this vigilance should include an environmental survey to anticipate changes in weather, wind direction, terrain, and daylight that can affect response and rescue efforts. This information should be communicated through incident command and helps to shape scene security and travel routes for emergency and rescue vehicles. Securing the scene and protecting individuals limits the overall spread of the mass casualty event. Workforce safety is discussed in greater detail in Chapter 6.

1.8.4 Assess Hazards

A close corollary to safeguarding an incident scene, as well as subsequent casualty care settings and facilities, is the *assessment of hazards* to identify and mitigate potential secondary events, whether intentionally sequential or as a consequence of the primary event. By gathering information about ongoing and emerging hazards, the risk for those at the scene and beyond can be significantly mitigated.[21] For example, following a terrorist event, the area should be assessed for additional (secondary) hazards, to include explosive devices, potential structural collapse, and exposed utilities. Other secondary hazards include environmental damage and debris, such as fallen trees and branches, as well as dangers of a large crowd surge that may result in additional casualties. As an example of the breadth of secondary hazards that can derive from a primary event, hazards secondary to an earthquake are listed in Table 1-3.

TABLE 1-3 Hazards Secondary to an Earthquake

Landslide
Building collapse
Bridge collapse
Hazardous material spill
Fire
Dam/levee failure
Water pollution
Tsunami (tidal wave)
Seiche ("tidal wave" in an enclosed body of water, such as a lake)
Train wreck
Mass car crash
Utility exposure

1.8.5 Support

To respond sufficiently to an incident scene or to casualty influx, a needs assessment (via informal information gathering or a formal assessment tool) must be conducted. By defining resource needs and determining resource availability (what currently exists), an analysis regarding surge *capacity* (resources available) and surge *capability* (resources operable) can be made and communicated through incident command. Available *support resources* include physical, institutional, social, and economic assets, as well as personnel with particular qualifications. While capacity is generally assessed on the basis of local resources, capability can be expanded as nonlocal (regional, national, and global) resources join response efforts. Ideally, an assessment of available resources is conducted as part of disaster preparedness and planning efforts based on communication among the various local response agencies and coordinated by the local emergency operations office. Surge capacity and capability are discussed further in Chapter 3.

Documentation of support resources that currently exist and are available to respond should be readily accessible. Even with preplanning, this type of accounting may not be available at the event locale. On-the-ground assessment of needed and available support may serve as a supplement to planning efforts or may be the only assessment available. Such an assessment should include options for available space given the current condition of infrastructure elements (eg, buildings, homes, transportation) and available stocks of essential resources, such as food, water, and medical supplies.

1.8.6   Triage and Treatment

Disaster triage differs significantly, in both goal and practice, from that typically conducted during normal routine operational periods in hospital settings. Daily triage involves matching individual patient needs to the highest level of care available, so that sicker and more seriously injured patients receive treatment first. During a disaster, the focus of care shifts from the individual patient to the population of casualties. There is a dynamic tension between scarce resources and casualty needs. As such, the focus moves from providing care to the sickest and most severely injured patients first, to providing care to casualties most likely to benefit, thus ensuring the highest number of survivors and the greatest good across all disaster casualties.[22,23] This practice of maximizing aggregate benefit, while minimizing additional casualties, ultimately diverts resources from the sickest and most injured to those most readily treatable and salvageable. Triage and treatment issues are discussed in greater detail in Chapters 2 and 7. Issues and challenges associated with the allocation of scare resources are described in Chapters 3 and 5.

Following most disasters, those most severely injured die immediately at the scene, while the majority of survivors do not sustain critical injuries requiring immediate care. The challenge of triage in this setting, therefore, is to assess and identify rapidly the small number of casualties with critical injuries and who are able to be saved with the limited resources available.[24]

One technique used by first responders when initially approaching a mass casualty disaster scene is the SALT triage system: **s**ort, **a**ssess, **l**ife-saving interventions, and **t**reatment/transport.[25] These steps include global sorting and initial grouping based on response to motor commands; assessing casualties based on the combination of *salvageable* injury severity and immediate threats to life; providing, basic life-saving interventions; and initiating prioritized transport to follow-on treatment settings. The critically injured are identified, and medical personnel intervene to address rapidly correctable, life-threatening conditions that could be remedied by opening an airway, decompressing a tension pneumothorax, applying pressure or tourniquets to stop bleeding, or injecting antidotes after a chemical nerve agent event. Rapid assessment of airway—breathing—circulation in a critically injured casualty may lead to a focus on stopping the bleeding as the first priority for intervention. To achieve the greatest good for the greatest number of salvageable individual casualties, treatment is phased over time; after the life-threatening issues are addressed, the rest of the evaluation and management for the individual casualty is deferred in favor of addressing the life-threatening issues of other casualties.

The principles of disaster triage in acute events differ little from one disaster to another (all-hazards approach), for which SALT triage is useful. However, triage management goals differ for large-scale bioevents, in which limitation of disease transmission is an essential goal. The SEIRV triage categories reflect this goal (SEIRV: Susceptible, Exposed, Infectious, Removed by death or illness recovery, or Vaccine protected), and are inextricably tied to population-based decisions necessary to control the infectious outbreak.[12] SEIRV triage is discussed further in Chapter 2.

1.8.7 Evacuation

Evacuation away from the scene can be done both before and after critical events. In those situations when a potentially devastating event can be predicted, and time allows (such as an impending hurricane), populations can be evacuated to safer areas. Particular attention should be given to special needs populations, to include shut-ins, disabled, children, and hospitalized patients. Following the event, casualties should be evacuated to designated casualty collection areas located safely away from the scene. Efficient evacuations for both casualties and the uninjured are defined by ingress and egress routes that preserve forward flows (and minimize counter flows) of traffic and that facilitate ground and air evacuation, depending on weather, terrain, situation, and vehicle availability. A common myth is that casualties are brought to health care facilities by emergency medical service responders in an organized response; the reality is that most casualties, who are "walking wounded," arrive at hospitals on their own.

Evacuation during and after a mass casualty event is intended to "decompress" the disaster area, thereby enabling identification of and intervention for the critically injured, and allowing search and rescue to progress.[26-28] An efficient evacuation system will include alternate care facilities, such as clinics, rehabilitation centers, schools, churches, and mobile response hospitals. Such options are discussed in Chapter 3.

1.8.8 Recovery

Recovery, which must be initated at the local level, is the often lengthy process of returning to a state of "normal function" that approximates what existed prior to the disaster. Sometimes, this means defining and adjusting to the "new normal." Recovery is a process necessary to minimize both the physical and psychosocial impacts on the affected population, and it draws on the resiliency of the community. Recovery begins in the short term with acute scene restoration and then

Excess Mortality and Hurricane Katrina

One year post-Katrina, the New Orleans citizenry alerted a fragile public health system that newspaper obituary reports seemed uncommonly high. A subsequent study confirmed that New Orleans had experienced a 47% increase in mortality over its pre-hurricane demographic baseline rates. That a nontraditional source identified the excess mortality was attributable to an antiquated and hurricane-disabled health information system in which disease and mortality went undetected. This emphasizes the critical importance of surveillance systems as an essential public health infrastructure.[8,9] Excess mortality resulted from a stressed health care delivery system, with notable gaps in primary and specialty care (eg, cancer and mental health).[10,11]

extends into the broader surrounding community. Recovery must be planned for in advance of a disaster, as part of the community's "all-hazards" planning process. Recovery strategies can be developed that include plans for business continuity, transportation alternatives, temporary shelters, provision of mental health services, and backup suppliers for power and water. The PRE- (planning and practice, resilience, and education and training)- DISASTER paradigm is an important reminder that recovery cannot be an afterthought—it is the goal of effective disaster response.

Recovery efforts, if appropriately undertaken, can actually lead to a rebuilt community at lower risk from future disaster events. Prior problems within the community that can be resolved through reconstruction include increased availablity of affordable housing, improved traffic flow, expanded green space, and modernization of public facilties.[29] Such improvements can support an increase in a community's level of resilience and, conversely, decrease its level of vulnerabilty. Further, lessons learned from recovery efforts can help to build response capacity for future events, while confining the impact of events to more managable proportions.[30]

1.9 SUMMARY

Large-scale disasters and public health emergencies shift the focus of health care and well-being from the individual to the affected population. It is important to understand the health consequences of disasters in terms of both direct impact from injury and indirect effects to public health; such direct and indirect mortality and morbidity can be measured. Management of these events requires a taxonomy that reflects the dimensions of natural, human systems failure, and conflict-based disasters, alone or in combination, and coordinated response over different phases of the events. Formally recognizing public health consequences in the taxonomy and management of disasters is a critical first step in this process. Minimizing adverse health outcomes requires cooperative efforts that cross traditional boundaries of health specialties, professions, and nationalities. The DISASTER paradigm enables a common framework for mass casualty and population-based disaster management across the clinical care, public health, and emergency response sectors. Disasters increase scrutiny on the capacity and capability of health systems to respond to the clinical and public health consequences, and varying degrees of strength, weakness, and risk are exposed. Ensuring effective disaster response, for all affected ages and populations, requires a new mindset and organizational transformation—it is not business as usual.

REFERENCES

1. Subbarao I, Lyznicki J, Hsu E, et al. A consensus-based educational framework and competency set for the discipline of disaster medicine and public health preparedness. *Disaster Med Public Health Prep.* 2008;2:57–68.

2. Burkle FM Jr. Public health emergencies, cancer, and the legacy of Katrina. *Prehosp Disaster Med.* 2007;22:291–292.

3. Burkle FM Jr. Complex public health emergencies. In: Koenig K, Schultz CH, eds. *Koenig and Schultz's Disaster Medicine.* Cambridge, England: Cambridge University Press; 2010.

4. Nelson C, Lurie N, Wasserman J, et al. Conceptualizing and defining public health emergency preparedness. *Am J Public Health.* 2007;97(suppl 1):S9–S11.

5. Koenig KL, Dinerman N, Kuehl AF. Disaster nomenclature—a functional impact approach: the PICE system. *Acad Emerg Med.* 1996;3:723–727.

6. Burkle FM Jr. Mass casualty management of a large-scale bioterrorist event: an epidemiological approach that shapes triage decisions. *Emerg Med Clin North Am.* 2002;20:409–436.

7. Burkle FM Jr, Greenough PG. Impact of public health emergencies on modern disaster taxonomy, planning, and response. *Disaster Med Public Health Prep.* 2008;2:192–199.

8. Stephens KU, Grew D, Chin K, et al. Excess mortality in the aftermath of Hurricane Katrina: a preliminary report. *Disaster Med Public Health Prep.* 2007;1:5–20.

9. Kanter R. Child mortality after Hurricane Katrina. *Disaster Med Public Health Prep.* 2010;4:62–65.

10. Edwards TO, Young RA, Lowe AF. Caring for a surge of Hurricane Katrina evacuees in primary care clinics. *Ann Fam Med.* 2007;5:170–174.

11. Joseph DA, Wingo PA, King JB, et al. Use of state cancer surveillance data to estimate the cancer burden in disaster affected areas: Hurricane Katrina, 2005. *Prehosp Disaster Med.* 2007;22:282–290.

12. Burkle FM Jr. Population-based triage management in response to surge-capacity requirements during a large-scale bioevent disaster. *Acad Emerg Med.* 2006;11:1118–1129.

13. Burkle FM Jr. Future humanitarian crises: challenges for practice, policy, and public health. *Prehosp Disaster Med.* 2010;25:191–198.

14. Exxon Valdez Oil Spill Trustee Council; http://www.evostc.state.ak.us/; accessed November 14, 2010.

15. Teich JM, Wagner MM, Mackenzie CF, Schafer KO. The informatics response in disaster, terrorism, and war. *JAMIA.* 2002;9:97–104.

16. Burkle FM, Hsu, EB, Loehr MC, et al. Definition and functions of health unified command and emergency operations centers for large-scale bioevent disasters within the existing ICS. *Disaster Med Public Health Prep.* 2007;1:135–141.

17. Bigley GA, Roberts KH. The incident command system: high-reliability organizing for complex and volatile task environments. *Acad Manage J.* 2001;44(6):1281–1299.

18. Buck DA, Trainor JE, Aguirre BE. A critical evaluation of the incident command system and NIMS. *J Homeland Security Emerg Manage.* 2006;3:1–27.

19. Hsu EB, Thomas TL, Bass EB, Whyne D, Kelen GD, Green GB. Healthcare worker competencies for disaster training. *BMC Med Educ.* 2006;6:19.

20. Cushman JC, Pachter HL, Beaton HL. Two New York City hospitals' surgical response to the September 11, 2001, terrorist attack in New York City. *J Trauma.* 2003;54:147–155.

21. Lavalla R, Stoffel S. *Blueprint for Community Emergency Management: A Text for Managing Emergency Operations.* Olympia, WA: Emergency Response Institute; 1983.

22. Vaetch RM. Disaster preparedness and triage: justice and the common good. *Mount Sinai J Med.* 2005;72:236–241.

23. Lanoix R, Wiener DE, Zayas V. Concepts in disaster triage in the wake of the World Trade Center terrorist attack. *Topics Emerg Med.* 2002;24:60–71.

24. Born CT, Briggs SM, Ciraulo DL, et al. Disasters and mass casualties: general principles of response and management. *J Am Acad Orthop Surg.* 2007;15:388–396.

25. Lerner EB, Schwartz RB, Coule PL, et al. Mass casualty triage: an evaluation of the data and development of a proposed national guideline. *Disaster Med Public Health Prep.* 2008;2 (1, suppl):S25–S34.

26. Briggs SM, Brinsfield KH. *Advanced Disaster Medical Response: Manual for Providers.* Boston, MA: Boston Harvard Medical International; 2003.

27. Grissom TE, Farmer JC. The provision of sophisticated critical care beyond the hospital: lessons from physiology and military experiences that apply to civil disaster medical response. *Crit Care Med.* 2005;33(1, suppl):S13–S21.

28. Lowe DW, Briggs SM. Planning for mass civilian casualties overseas: IMSuRT – International Medical/Surgical Response Teams. *Clin Orthop Relat Res.* 2004;422:109–113.

29. Berke PR, Kartez J, Wenger D. Recovery after disaster: achieving sustainable development, mitigation, and equity. *Disasters.* 1993;17:1–8.

30. Adger WN, Hughes TP, Folke C, Carpenter SR, Rockström J. Social-ecological resilience to coastal disasters. *Science.* 2005;309:1036–1039.

CHAPTER TWO

Triage for Disasters and Public Health Emergencies

E. Brooke Lerner, PhD

Jim Lyznicki, MS, MPH

Italo Subbarao, DO, MBA

Frederick M. Burkle, Jr., MD, MPH, DTM

Arthur Cooper, MD, MS

John H. Armstrong, MD

2.1 PURPOSE

This chapter describes triage schemes that may be utilized during a disaster or public health emergency. Mass casualty triage is used for an event that occurs in a limited geographic location (eg, an explosion or building collapse), and population-based triage is needed when an expanding event generates casualties who are distributed across a wider geography (eg, pandemic or flood). A single event may become a disaster that requires both mass casualty and population-based triage.

2.2 LEARNING OBJECTIVES

After completing this chapter, readers will be able to:

➤ Articulate the purpose and rationale for mass casualty triage.

➤ Discuss the elements of effective pre-hospital and hospital triage.

➤ Describe the challenges associated with mass casualty triage, including over- and under-triage.

➤ Explain the purpose and rationale for population-based triage.

2.3   DISASTER MEDICINE AND PUBLIC HEALTH PREPAREDNESS COMPETENCIES ADDRESSED[1]

➤ Explain the strengths and limitations of various triage systems that have been developed for the management of mass casualties at a disaster scene or receiving facility. (5.1.2)

➤ Perform mass casualty triage at a disaster scene or receiving facility. (5.1.3)

➤ Develop, evaluate, and revise mass casualty and population-based triage policies, protocols, and procedures that may be implemented in a disaster or public health emergency. (5.1.5)

2.4   INTRODUCTION

All disasters, regardless of cause, have similarities in their clinical and public health consequences. The events differ in the degree to which these consequences affect the population and disrupt the clinical and public health infrastructure in the affected region. When events become disasters, emergency needs at the scene and at local health care facilities overwhelm local resources. To save the most lives possible, available resources must be used as efficiently as possible. Formal triage schemes are used to guide emergency responders and health care facilities in making casualty decisions based on resource availability. By using a formalized triage system, the decision of who should receive resources first is more objective and reproducible. Triage has two components: (1) sorting casualties and prioritizing their care on the basis of the severity of injuries and illnesses and (2) optimizing the allocation of available resources by directing those resources to casualties who are most likely to benefit.

For events that occur in a defined geographic region, numerous tools have been developed to help sort casualties into a few large categories. This allows responders to quickly identify the group of casualties who need immediate intervention and subsequent transport. However, during a large event, the number of casualties who are identified as needing immediate aid may still be larger than the number of resources available to care for them. In this case, casualties will need to be further prioritized within each category. For events that involve a wider geography and a sizeable percentage of the population, whether injured, ill, or simply at risk, population-based triage is needed to contain risk within communities and maximize return from available resources.

2.5   MASS CASUALTY TRIAGE

Recent examples of events that emphasize the need to sort casualties include the Madrid (2004), London (2005), and Moscow (2010) train bombings; the Virginia Tech shootings (2007); and the Minneapolis bridge collapse (2007).

For instance, the Madrid train bombings generated more than 2000 casualties; the local response system was quickly overwhelmed and had to prioritize casualties for treatment and transport.[2] Mass casualty triage is used any time there are more casualties than responders, whether for a few minutes or for the entire response. A single responder at a car crash with three occupants may use mass casualty triage principles to decide who to care for first, yet as additional responders arrive on scene, all injured people will begin to receive care, and mass casualty triage will no longer be used.

Mass casualty events (MCEs) are likely to involve a mix of critical and non-critically injured casualties, skewed toward the latter. Non-critically injured casualties will likely survive without rapid interventions; thus, the mass casualty triage system should focus on minimizing morbidity and mortality of the critically injured. Because resources are overwhelmed and insufficient to maximize treatment to each individual casualty, the goal in response changes from the greatest good for the individual to the greatest good for the greatest number of casualties. This means not only prioritizing casualties for treatment, but also recognizing those casualties with limited survivability even with maximal resources. Under these circumstances, resources are better used on other casualties with greater likelihood of survival.

Within the first hours of a disaster, mass casualty triage is usually performed by local first responders, emergency response personnel, and health care facility first receivers. Ideally, casualties will be rapidly categorized away from the scene by the most experienced medical personnel available to identify the level of care that is needed. Comprehension of the basic medical consequences of various injuries (eg, blast, crush, and burns injuries, and exposure to chemical, biologic, and radioactive agents) across all demographics in the community (eg, children, elderly) is critical.

The challenge faced by responders is that not all casualties can be seen at once. A systematic method is needed to decide rapidly which casualties need urgent interventions and which casualties do not. This shift in mindset is difficult—it is only natural to try to do everything for everyone. However, the outcome of this thinking is likely a higher mortality rate.

The science related to mass casualty triage is limited. In general, most work has focused on the initial sorting of casualties into priority categories. When an incident is large, the group of casualties categorized as the first priority for care may still be too large to be immediately treated or transported with the available resources, and additional assessments will need to be made to further prioritize those who have the most immediate needs. An effective triage system should be an iterative process that reduces error through sequential casualty and resource assessments across all settings of casualty care. Triage should separate the critically injured immediate casualties from the much larger group of non-critically injured casualties.

2.5.1   Initial Sorting of Casualties

The most basic initial triage method is sorting the living casualties from those obviously dead. Further assessment of casualty need focuses on threats to life, limb, and eyesight, as well as the survivability of injuries. It is recommended that a mass casualty triage system be used to guide these decisions so that they are more likely to be objective and reproducible. In an ideal world, mass casualty triage will occur at the scene or at a casualty collection point. The reality from numerous real-world events is that many casualties self-transport to health care facilities away from, yet in proximity to, the scene. Thus, personnel at health care facilities need to be familiar with mass casualty triage.

Mass casualty triage protocols are used to prioritize casualties in the field for treatment, evacuation, and transport for further care. These systems prioritize casualties into categories, typically immediate, delayed, minimal, expectant, and dead. Interventions for immediately life-threatening conditions can be performed as identified during the triage process. These interventions should be simple procedures that can be performed rapidly and under conditions of rescuer/responder and casualty safety.

The National Disaster Life Support™ (NDLS™) Program encourages the use of the SALT (**s**ort, **a**ssess, **l**ifesaving interventions, and **t**reatment/transport) triage method for mass casualty triage; however, providers should be familiar with the mass casualty triage system that is used in their community.[3]

2.5.1.1 SALT Triage

SALT triage was designed as a proposed national guideline for primary mass casualty triage.[3] It is simple to use and easy to remember. It instructs providers to quickly *sort* casualties by their ability to follow commands, individually *assess* casualties and apply *lifesaving interventions* rapidly, and assign a *treatment and/or transport* priority. SALT triage was developed by a consensus review panel, based on the best scientific evidence available. SALT triage includes these core concepts:[3]

➤ Voice commands to sort casualties at the scene.

➤ Interventions including controlling hemorrhage, opening airway, decompressing the chest (for tension pneumothorax), and autoinjecting antidotes for chemical injury.

➤ Separation of expectant casualties from the dead. Identification of expectant casualties is based on available resources.

➤ Simple application for casualties of any age and from any type of mass casualty incident.

Initial clinical studies of SALT triage demonstrate a higher accuracy rate than those published for other triage systems while accomplished with a similar speed.[4]

SALT triage is accomplished in two steps: global sorting and individual assessment (Figure 2-1).

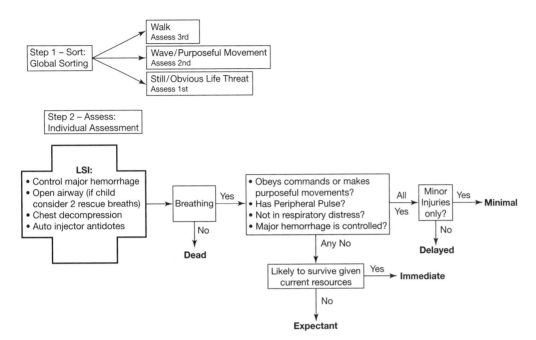

FIGURE 2-1
SALT Mass Casualty
Triage[3]

Source: Lerner EB, Schwartz RB, Coule PL, Weinstein ES, Cone DC, Hunt RC, et al. Mass casualty triage: an evaluation of the data and development of a proposed national guideline. Disaster Med and Public Health Prep. 2008;2(Suppl 1): S25–S34.

Step 1: global sorting.   The outcome of global sorting is to separate the minimally injured casualties, who are least likely to require emergent care, from the rest of the casualty population. These casualties are awake and ambulatory. They are identified by instructing, "Everyone who can hear me and who needs medical attention, please move to [a designated area]." The location to which these ambulatory casualties are directed must be safe and have some visible element of care. Their ability to walk indicates that they are likely to have (1) intact airway, breathing, and circulation and (2) intact mental status, at least to the extent that they can follow commands. These casualties are the third priority for individual assessment.

If the objective of triage is to find the critically injured, it may seem paradoxical to invest time upfront for identification of the minimally injured. However, this group can be a significant distraction from the smaller number of critically injured. Active management of the minimally injured may redirect self-transports and reduce the burden of minimally injured casualties flooding the closest hospitals. This can save limited hospital resources for the more critically ill.

It is important to remember that this process will not be perfect: casualties with critical injuries may be assisted or carried by other casualties or bystanders to a designated non-critical area, or casualties who are able to walk may have injury progression, necessitating more urgent care. Thus, casualties who can walk should be individually assessed and should not be assumed to have minimal injuries.

The next group identified includes those casualties who cannot walk, but are awake and able to follow the commands. They are identified by stating to the remaining casualties, "Everyone who can hear me, please raise an arm or a leg so that we can come help you." This group is individually assessed second. Airway, breathing, circulation, and mental status in these casualties are at least adequate to allow them to follow simple commands. However, since they are not ambulatory, they may have mild hypotension, mild hypoxemia, or significant musculoskeletal injuries.

The remaining casualties are those who neither walk nor wave, and remain still. These are prioritized first for individual assessment and fall into three groups: critically injured/salvageable, unsalvageable, and dead.

Step 2: individual assessment. The next step in SALT triage is to assess each individual casualty and perform simple lifesaving interventions as indicated. Individual assessment also assigns casualties to a triage category, which links casualty needs with priority for treatment and transport to the next level of care. The goal of this step is to provide immediate lifesaving interventions to the critically injured/salvageable. It should be remembered that sorting is an imperfect process, and critically injured/salvageable casualties may be assigned to noncritical groups; it should never be assumed that the groups are completely accurate. Reassessment can enhance accuracy and reduce errors.

The temptation in an MCE is to assess and manage casualties as "patients," trying to do more of what is done routinely in the emergency medical response to traumatic injuries. MCEs are different, and "business as usual" does not apply. Four simple lifesaving interventions have been identified that can be applied quickly with minimal resources, do not require a responder to stay with the casualty, and are likely to reduce morbidity and mortality:

➤ *Controlling major hemorrhage* can be done by using tourniquets or by having another person or device provide direct pressure.

➤ *Opening the airway* should be done only with simple positioning maneuvers such as chin lift/jaw thrust or with insertion of a basic airway adjunct (oropharyngeal, nasopharyngeal). If the casualty is a child who is not breathing, two rescue breaths should be considered.

➤ *Decompressing the chest with a needle* should be done for tension pneumothorax.

➤ *Autoinjecting nerve agent antidotes* should be done for symptomatic nerve agent casualties.

These lifesaving interventions are performed if appropriate equipment is readily available and the interventions are within the provider's competence, can be performed quickly (less than a minute), and do not require the provider to remain with the casualty.

After consideration of lifesaving interventions, each casualty is assigned a triage category by following a stepwise process. The color-coded triage categories include immediate (red), delayed (yellow), minimal (green), expectant (gray), and dead (black). The provider starts by determining whether the casualty is breathing. If not breathing after an attempt to open the airway, then the person is dead and the provider proceeds to the next casualty. If the casualty is a child, two rescue breaths may be attempted, but if the child is still not breathing, then he or she is dead. The differential intervention between adult and pediatric casualty respiratory arrest reflects the different nature of respiratory arrest between these two casualty populations.

If the casualty is breathing, yet is unable to obey commands or make purposeful movements, has no palpable peripheral pulse, is in respiratory distress, or has uncontrolled external hemorrhage, then the provider should consider the likelihood of the casualty's survival given available resources. If likely to survive, then the casualty is categorized as immediate. Immediate casualties are critically injured with the most serious, yet potentially survivable life-threatening injuries. If unlikely to survive, then the casualty is categorized as expectant.

Expectant casualties are still alive, but are so severely injured they have little chance of survival either absolutely (eg, 100% body surface area burns) or relatively given the available resources. During a mass casualty incident, resources will initially not be available to care for expectant casualties. As additional resources become available, resuscitation should be attempted or comfort care should be provided. It bears emphasis that the expectant group is heterogeneous; some casualties are absolutely unsalvageable under the best of circumstances, and some are relatively unsalvageable given the scarce resources. As resources become available, expectant casualties in the relatively unsalvageable category may be moved to the immediate category.

If the casualty is able to follow commands or make purposeful movements, has peripheral pulses, is not in respiratory distress, and does not have a life-threatening external hemorrhage, then the casualty category is either minimal (requiring minor care and will not deteriorate if care is delayed indefinitely) or delayed (requiring further definitive care, such as fracture fixation, but will not deteriorate if care is delayed for a defined interval). This assessment can be more subjective but, in general, rests on whether the casualty could receive no initial care without an increased risk of morbidity or mortality.

Casualties should be visually marked with their assigned triage category by applying a triage tag, physically moving them to an area designated for their triage category, or writing on the casualty's skin with permanent marker. The last of these is simple and effective. In some cases, a combination of methods may be useful. It is important to consider that casualty tags can become damaged or lost, and that there have been reports of casualties "gaming the system" by changing their tag. Areas for grouping can be designated with large, colored tarps or flags.

During this process, dead casualties should not be moved unless they are obstructing access to other casualties. This will preserve any evidence that might be useful to law enforcement investigators; excessive manipulation of human remains may destroy relevant evidence. Even for noncriminal incidents, it is important to limit strain on immediate resources by deferring movement of the dead until appropriate resources arrive.

2.5.1.2   Other Mass Casualty Triage Systems

Other mass casualty triage systems vary considerably, from clinical assessment only to the use of physiologic parameters to prioritize casualties. A brief description of existing systems is provided in Table 2-1.[5-11]

TABLE 2-1   Comparison of Existing Primary Mass Casualty Triage Systems Adapted from Lerner et al[3]

System	Coding	Basis of Status Assignment	Therapies Before Assigning Dead Category	Comments
Simple Triage and Rapid Treatment (START)[5]	Immediate: red Delayed: yellow Walking wounded: green Deceased: black	Immediate: cannot follow commands, respiratory rate >30, slow capillary refill Walking wounded: able to walk Deceased: not breathing after 1 airway attempt Delayed: all other casualties	1 airway attempt through positioning	*No palpable radial pulse* replaces *capillary refill* in modified version
CareFlight[6]	Immediate (red) Urgent (yellow) Delayed (green) Unsalvageable (black)	Immediate: does not follow commands, no palpable radial pulse Urgent: does not walk but obeys commands and has radial pulse Delayed: walks Unsalvageable: not breathing with open airway	Open airway	Does not consider respiratory rate Used for adults or children
CESIRA[3]	Red Yellow Green	Red: unconscious, bleeding, in shock, insufficient breathing Yellow: none of the above with broken bones or other injuries Green: able to walk	None	No dead category: only physician can declare death in Italy Based on presenting problem Name is based on order conditions are evaluated
JumpSTART[7]	Immediate (red) Delayed (yellow) Minor (green) Deceased (black)	Immediate: respiratory rate <15, >45 or irregular, no palpable peripheral pulse, inappropriate posturing (P) or unresponsive (U) on the AVPU scale	Open airway using basic positioning; if there is still no breathing and there is palpable radial pulse, give 5 rescue breaths.	Developed for pediatric casualties 1–8 years old Developed to parallel structure of START triage system

TABLE 2-1 *(Continued)*

		Delayed: unable to walk, regular respiratory rate 15–45, palpable peripheral pulse, alert (A) or verbal (V) on the AVPU scale Minor: able to walk Dead: not breathing after 1 attempt to open airway and 5 rescue breaths	Reassess after immediate and delayed children have received care	Children carried to ambulatory area should be the first assessed in that area Has modification for nonambulatory children
Homebush[8]	Immediate (red) Urgent (yellow/gold) Not urgent (green) Dying (white) Dead (black) Also assigned radio voice categories: Immediate (Alpha) Urgent (Bravo) Not urgent (Charlie) Dying (Delta) Dead (Echo)	Not urgent: anyone who can walk Dead: not breathing Dying: casualties assessed as being beyond help Immediate: not walking, breathing but not able to follow commands, no radial pulse, respiratory rate >30 Urgent: nonambulatory casualties who do not meet other criteria	One attempt to open airway using basic positioning methods	Based on START and SAVE triage Category for dying created so they can receive comfort care Uses geographic triage with flags rather than individual triage tags
Military triage[9]	Immediate Delayed Minor Expectant	Immediate: those who should be treated first, with list of possible injuries Delayed: those who can have a delay of 6-8 hours before treatment Minor: those who will not have significant mortality if no further care is provided Expectant: those with signs of impending death or who require vast resources for treatment	Open airway	Secondary triage includes system for casualty evacuation Colors used to mark casualties can vary across nations

(Continued)

TABLE 2-1 *(Continued)*

System	Coding	Basis of Status Assignment	Therapies Before Assigning Dead Category	Comments
Pediatric triage tape (PTT)[10]	Immediate (red) Urgent (yellow) Delayed (green) Dead	Immediate: abnormally slow or fast respiratory rate *or* abnormally slow or fast pulse rate Urgent: not walking with capillary refill <2 seconds Delayed: Child who is walking *or* infant who is alert and moving all limbs Dead: Not breathing	Does not breathe after airway is opened by jaw thrust	Requires tape that uses height to show providers age-appropriate parameters to triage child (4 sizes of children: 50–80, 80–100, 100–140, and >140 cm) Adaptation of triage SIEVE
Sacco triage method (STM)[11]	Group 1 (high rate of deterioration) Group 2 (moderate) Group 3 (slow)	Assigns an "RPM" score based on respiratory rate (R), pulse (P), and motor response (M)	Score = 0 for no vital signs Before scoring, open airway, decompress pneumothorax, stop bleeding	Provides score for each casualty Grouping of casualties changes with availability of resources Transport order by score, not group
Triage SIEVE[12,13]	Priority 1 (immediate): Red Priority 2 (urgent): yellow Priority 3 (delayed): green Priority 4 (expectant): blue Dead: white or black	Priority 1: not walking with respiratory rate <10 or >29 *or* capillary refill >2 seconds Priority 2: not walking with respiratory rate 10–29 *and* capillary refill <2 seconds Priority 3: walking Dead: no airway	Open airway	Heart rate >120 is substituted for capillary refill in cold conditions or poor light Does not use mental status

2.5.2   Treatment and Transport After Mass Casualty Triage

In an MCE, mass casualty triage is used to establish the order in which casualties receive care and/or transport. In some situations, it may be necessary to refine casualty prioritization near the disaster scene within the five assigned triage categories. For instance, five people who need immediate care may be identified but only two transport units may be available. As a result, those five casualties will need to be further prioritized to identify who will be transported by the two available units and who will wait.

The triage category defines a treatment/transport priority: immediate casualties are the first priority, followed by delayed, minimal, and expectant casualties. While this sequence is logical, lucid casualties may behave in their own self-interest and not wait near the scene for organized transport. For those needing transport, efficient use of transport assets may include mixing categories of triaged persons and using alternate forms of transport (eg, buses) to move minimally injured casualties away from the scene more quickly and efficiently.

This is an area where limited work has been done to give providers guidance on how to proceed. Several instruments have been developed but have not been well studied. The US military uses "evacuation priority" categories to prioritize the transport of triaged casualties. This system is subjective and is based on clinical assessment to assign a predicted time interval during which a casualty may decompensate. Military evacuation priorities include urgent, priority, and routine. Urgent evacuation casualties are those who should be evacuated within two hours to save life, limb, or eyesight. Priority casualties are those who should be evacuated within four hours because of concern for casualty deterioration beyond that point. Routine casualties are those whose condition is not expected to worsen significantly and who will require evacuation within the next 24 hours. This system is most commonly used in armed conflicts; there is very limited information on its use in the civilian setting. Further, it creates only three categories of casualties, and in a large event further prioritization may still be needed within these categories.

The SAVE (**S**econdary **A**ssessment of **V**ictim **E**ndpoint) triage and triage SORT methods have been developed in the civilian sector in an attempt to provide prehospital personnel with more detailed guidelines for assigning treatment priorities. The SAVE triage instrument was designed for mass casualty events in which providers have limited medical resources to treat casualties at the disaster site and when evacuation to definitive care will be prolonged.[5] Similar to the military evacuation priorities, SAVE categorizes casualties into three groups: (1) those who will die regardless of the care they receive, (2) those who will survive regardless of the care they receive, and (3) those who will benefit significantly from field interventions. The SAVE algorithm assesses casualty survivability by describing the relationship between expected benefits and resources consumed, using trauma statistics. Preexisting disease and age are factored into SAVE triage decisions.[5] Similarly, the SORT triage method categorizes casualties based on a physiologic score calculated by the Triage Revised Trauma Score.[14] The score is used to place casualties into three priority groups or categorize them as dead.

Clearly, the importance of prioritizing casualties within the mass casualty triage categories increases as the number of casualties increases and the availability of resources decreases. Clinical judgment will be necessary to help guide these decisions even if one of the described formal systems is used. Further, the more complex the triage system, the more difficult it will be to execute during a mass casualty event.

2.5.3 Hospital Triage

Hospital management includes efforts to meet the needs of acutely ill or injured casualties through rapid evaluation and stabilization until definitive care is available. This includes clinical considerations for critical casualties, casualty redistribution to alternate care sites, and the evacuation of health care facilities. Triage is dynamic across the hospital. Casualty flow is regulated by section chiefs at control points in the emergency department, operating room, intensive care unit, ward, and radiology department. Section chiefs should reassess casualties regularly.

Hospitals must have triage systems to cope with potential incidents in proximity to their facility, where a large number of casualties can present without warning before an emergency medical services response has been initiated. Casualties with relatively minor problems may arrive before those with serious conditions, thus inundating the emergency department and occupying valuable beds. Casualties may also arrive at the hospital without being triaged or having received stabilizing medical treatment. Difficulties usually arise not from a lack of resources, but from a failure in coordination of resources. A practiced incident management system works to synchronize resource utilization.[15]

Hospitals need to integrate the care of normal daily emergency patients, the number of whom may increase because of psychological, cardiac, and respiratory problems exacerbated by the event, with the care of casualties from the event. Patients with chronic diseases may create additional strain on acute care resources when the outpatient services on which these patients depend for management of their chronic disease are disrupted by the event.

Many hospital plans assume that the majority of casualties are critically injured. Across hazards, the reality is that most casualties are not critically injured. This fact reflects the lethality of disasters. It is estimated that approximately 20% of casualties will be critically injured.[15] The triage challenge at the hospital is to sift through all of the casualties, the majority of whom are not critically injured, to find the smaller number of casualties who are critically injured.

Of the 20% of casualties who are critically injured, it is likely that less than a quarter (5% of all casualties) will need an emergency operation. Up to half (10% of all casualties) may be re-categorized as delayed after initial intervention. Delayed casualties need monitoring to detect injury progression that results in immediate needs.[15]

Setting conditions for success in finding the critically injured requires staffed care areas for "minimal" and "expectant" casualties, not in the emergency department and preferably out of the hospital. The expectant area must be separate from the morgue; expectant patients are alive and need comfort care, as well as reassessment in light of resource availability over time.

Interventions are guided by the "crisis standard of care" used in the disaster context. Applying the principle of "greatest good for the greatest number," phased interventions are performed. This means that casualty assessments and interventions are extended over a longer time interval than in non-disaster situations. Thus, more acute interventions can be performed across the casualty population to keep more casualties alive. The goal is optimal care for the casualty population (rather than the daily optimal care for every patient). The phases include:

➤ Lifesaving interventions/primary survey (fixing broken vital signs).

➤ Secondary survey (clinical determination of anatomic injuries).

➤ Radiologic survey (radiographic determination of anatomic injuries).

➤ Tertiary survey (reassessment of physiology, anatomy, and studies).

In non-MCEs, the first three phases are usually completed within an hour; in an MCE, they may be extended over hours to days.

Special triage situations can arise when hospital resources either are damaged or have to be abandoned during an incident. Staffing shortages can suddenly arise as health care workers spontaneously evacuate the facility in anticipation of a hazard or cannot reach the hospital because of transportation problems.

2.5.4   Challenges and Pitfalls

Mass casualty triage is an imperfect process implemented under difficult and austere conditions. It is a dynamic process that is constantly influenced by changes in casualty needs, scene conditions, resource availability, and time. Effective triage depends on quick clinical assessments, situational awareness, and rapid decision making.

Mass casualty triage is unique in that there are large numbers of injured or ill persons to be prioritized, with significantly fewer care providers than there are casualties. These providers are typically further constrained by an infrastructure and system that is insufficient to handle the number of casualties: there is limited equipment at the scene, transport capabilities are not sufficient for the number of casualties, and hospital resources are stretched so that alternative destinations or facilities outside the typical response area need to be considered. Providers also are faced with potential personal and casualty risks, such as the possibility of contamination, requiring appropriate personal protective equipment and decontamination capability, and the presence of secondary hazards. Finally, because of the overwhelming number of casualties and resource needs, multiple agencies will need to work together in response efforts. This requires a common language and a common understanding of what steps need to be taken for an effective response.

Triage systems are resource-dependent, and the health and emergency management systems must allow for dynamic triage decisions based on changes in available resources and casualty needs. In an MCE, resources and personnel may become depleted or increasingly available as the situation evolves.

Mass casualty triage should be used to allocate or ration resources only when the system is overwhelmed. Otherwise, triage should be based on physiologic priority: casualties with threats to their airways are managed before those with threats to their breathing and circulation. Providers can expect the system to begin to break down when critical casualty load per hour exceeds five patients, and to become wholly chaotic when casualty load per hour approaches 20 patients.[16]

Triage is dynamic and reflects a casualty's condition and available resources at the time of assessment. All casualties should be periodically reassessed and retriaged, as time, conditions, and resources permit. The importance of frequent, individual reevaluation by trained medical personnel is that triage accuracy increases. Individual casualty triage categorization should be adjusted to reflect changes. Casualties initially assigned to the minimal group, for example, may show signs of previously unrecognized illness or injury and may need to be upgraded to a more urgent category. In the chaotic circumstances of mass casualty triage, mistakes will occur; casualty reassessment enables an error-tolerant system and overcomes human fallibility.[15]

Effective triage requires a balance between the demands on the system and the supply of resources in a way that minimizes undertriage and overtriage.

Over-triage assigns non-critically injured casualties to a higher triage category. Thus, the true critically injured are diluted by non-critically injured casualties, and scarce resources are applied to casualties who do not need them at that time. Over-triage is associated with an increased overall critical mortality rate,[15] as shown in Figure 2-2.[17]

FIGURE 2-2

Relationship of Over-triage Rate to Critical Mortality Rate in 14 Terrorist Events[15]

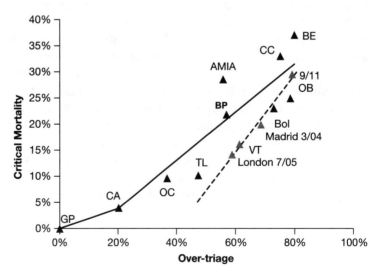

Dotted line represents recent (last decade) terrorist attacks. GP, Guildford pubs; CA, Craigavon; OC, Oklahoma City; TL, Tower of London; BP, Birmingham pubs; Bol, Bologna; AMIA, Buenos Aires; OB, Old Bailey; CC, Cu Chi; BE, Beirut; VT, Virginia Tech.

Under-triage assigns critically injured casualties to a lower triage category. This occurs when the severity of casualty illness or injury is unrecognized and results in delayed treatment. This leads to an increase in the critical mortality rate of the casualty population, as well as an increase in the risk of death of the under-triaged individual casualty.

Assessment of triage schemes should include determinations of the over-triage and under-triage rates. SALT triage has been found in simulated disaster scenarios to have an under-triage rate between 4% and 11% and an over-triage rate between 8% and 14%.[4,18]

Critical decision making and outcomes are only as good as the underlying triage management system. Accordingly, triage management cannot be thought of as an isolated agency-, department-, or hospital-level process. The seamless integration of a systems-based framework, coordinated through the incident command system, can help ensure that treatment prioritizations are undertaken in a manner that is effective and equitable (see Chapter 4).[18]

Select triage performance pitfalls are outlined in Table 2-2 and can be overcome with triage drills using a uniform mass casualty triage system.

TABLE 2-2 10 Pitfalls in Triage

Pre-hospital	Hospital
Focusing on casualties, to the exclusion of scene considerations	Letting non-critical casualties into hospital
Seeing casualty population as group of individual patients	Performing history and physical, rather than physiologic screen on each casualty
Letting severe anatomic injuries distract from physiologic screen	Not using expectant category
Expecting walking wounded to stay at the scene	Not performing sequential triage (reassessment over time)
Performing more than essential life-saving interventions	Using radiographs in initial casualty assessment

2.6 POPULATION-BASED TRIAGE

Triage decision making for widespread disasters and public health emergencies, whether from a natural disaster, pandemic, or human-caused event, differs from mass casualty triage because there are large numbers of casualties distributed across a larger area and the population as a whole remains at risk from the event. The management perspective thus broadens to include not only affected casualties, but the entire at-risk community. Thus, available resources must be used to achieve the greatest good for the greatest number of casualties *and* for the entire population. Reducing casualty morbidity and mortality, as well as the preventable morbidity and mortality in the general population, becomes the goal.

2.6.1   Population-Based Triage Methods for Biologic Events

Triage decisions for populations affected by biologic events are based on inter-related information including illness severity, infectiousness, and duration of illness. Experience with the severe acute respiratory syndrome (SARS) outbreak in 2003 demonstrated the value of population-based triage that allowed for prioritization of groups most in need of intervention while recognizing the need to limit disease transmission to the at-risk community. In general, the goal of population triage for a biologic event is to protect casualties with the disease *and* the susceptible population who are currently not infected with the disease.[19]

Conventional MCE triage is based on severity of illness or injury and does not consider additional elements, such as exposure, duration, or infectiousness. Thus, population triage during a biologic event assigns a priority to treatment while attempting to prevent secondary transmission through the implementation of nonmedical strategies (eg, social distancing, shelter-in-place, isolation, quarantine, risk communication) and medical interventions (eg, immunization, prophylactic medication, respiratory support). The mnemonic SEIRV can be used to categorize members of the community during a biologic event. It defines five categories of people and can be used to prevent secondary disease transmission:[19]

➤ **S**usceptible: people who are not yet exposed but are susceptible.

➤ **E**xposed: people who are susceptible and have been in contact with an infected person; they may be infected but are not yet contagious.

➤ **I**nfectious: casualties who are symptomatic and contagious.

➤ **R**emoved: casualties who no longer can transmit the disease to others because they have survived and developed immunity or died from the disease.

➤ **V**accinated (or medicated): people who have received prophylactic medical intervention to protect them from infection.

With a biologic event, everyone in the affected population will fall into one of the five SEIRV categories; two categories (infectious and removed) cover the acutely ill and recovering casualties, and three categories (susceptible, exposed, and vaccinated) cover the remaining population. Effective community response must identify exposed and infectious populations, separate them from the unexposed yet susceptible general population, and manage each triage category in ways that limit spread. Risk communication strategies can work for the susceptible, exposed, and vaccinated categories. The prehospital and hospital responses must focus on taking appropriate precautions when treating the infectious and removed (yet still ill) groups. For example, transporting an unexposed and very anxious individual to a hospital under the circumstances of a biologic event will actually expose that individual to the infection. Alternatives include transport to a nonhospital acute care facility that has not treated any infected individuals and provision of information to that individual regarding risk factors for infection.[19]

2.6.2   Population-Based Triage Through Risk Communication

Effective risk communication informs members of the affected community about how to reduce the risk of exposure and about how and where to access care if needed. By providing proactive and accurate information, health and emergency response agencies can better manage the population's demand for services. Collaboration in risk communication between health care facilities, emergency management, and public safety organizations is critical and enhances community situational awareness.

Getting accurate information to people quickly is a key component to saving lives during any emergency. Most disaster management failures are related to communication shortfalls. Crisis and emergency risk communication provides information for individuals, stakeholders, or an entire community to support the best possible decisions to protect their own health. During emergencies, the public may receive information from a variety of sources. Effective communication of clear, concise, and credible information will help assure the public that the situation is being addressed competently. Public information must reach broad audiences to publicize both immediate and anticipated health hazards, appropriate health and safety precautions, the need for evacuation through alternative travel routes, the proper indications and venues for seeking medical attention, distribution or dispensing sites, and sheltering.

In 2003, the Canadian experience with the outbreak of SARS improved community management by demonstrating the beneficial use of disease-specific telephone hotlines and call centers to assist the population in determining potential exposure risks, the need for medical attention, and the best places to seek care. Hotlines helped assure people of the benefits of social distancing and the benefits of remaining at home when clinical treatment was unnecessary. In 2009, this strategy was employed by various communities worldwide to address the H1N1 influenza pandemic. Experience with H1N1 hotlines in both New Zealand and China showed a measurable improvement in the number of callers who chose self-care over a visit to the hospital emergency department after speaking with hotline operators.[20]

In a serious infectious disease outbreak, people will share a common concern: they will want to know whether they have been exposed and are possibly infectious, or unexposed and thus susceptible. Counter intuitively, the latter category routinely requires the most attention and educational resources. Risk communication should be directed toward helping local residents determine their risk status and take actions to protect themselves and others from disease spread. In other events, like a flood, risk communication should include information on how to address basic human needs (eg, where to get food or water, or where to go for shelter), as well as self protection (eg, how to prevent mold, risks associated with swimming/walking through flood waters).

2.6.3   Population-Based Triage at the Regional Level

Some events will have a large and prolonged health burden, and system-wide triage decisions must be made on the basis of data collection and analysis. These events have the potential to require emergency mass critical care for a significant number of casualties over a prolonged period.

In the United States, a core societal expectation is nearly limitless provision of health care to those who want it, especially with acute illness and injury. Provision of health care during disasters challenges this expectation. When efforts to augment health care are insufficient to meet demands, and there is no fair and just system to allocate scarce life-sustaining interventions, then community trust in the broader health care delivery system may be lost, thereby compromising the entire medical and public health response. A regional approach will be needed that focuses on regional resource allocation and promotes transparency and situational awareness across the region.[21] One model for management of regional resources is the regional Health Emergency Operations Center (HEOC), discussed further in Chapter 4. The HEOC consolidates population health care decisions within the incident command system.

Triage decisions at the regional level affect the allocation of scarce resources, to include pharmaceutical stockpiles and vaccines; redistribution of physical and human resources within the affected region; and implementation of emergency mass critical care provisions and protocols, such as the use of the Sequential Organ Failure Assessment (SOFA) score for admission to intensive care units and the allocation of ventilators.[22] Acknowledgement of crisis standards of care would facilitate these decisions.

2.6.4   Population-Based Triage and Allocation of Critical Care Resources

Multiple groups have attempted to address the allocation of medical resources in response to a prolonged public health emergency, such as a nuclear detonation or an influenza pandemic. The Ontario Protocol (2006) represents a seminal approach in this area and was based on reflection regarding the SARS epidemic. This protocol can be used for any event in which critical care resources may be overwhelmed. The protocol establishes three criteria through which critical care resource allocation can be determined for each casualty: inclusion, exclusion, and minimum qualifications of survival (MQS). Inclusion criteria are focused on the traditional requirements for invasive ventilator support and for management of severe shock. The exclusion criteria are listed in Table 2-3 and catalog situations associated with very poor outcomes.[23]

TABLE 2-3 Exclusion Criteria for Ventilator Access[23]

➤ Cardiac arrest: unwitnessed arrest, recurrent arrest, arrest unresponsive to standard measures; trauma-related arrest.

➤ Metastatic malignancy with poor prognosis.

➤ Severe burn: body surface area >40%, severe inhalation injury.

➤ End-stage organ failure:

  ➢ Cardiac: New York Heart Association class III or IV.

  ➢ Pulmonary: severe chronic lung disease with FEV_1* <25%.

  ➢ Hepatic: MELD** score >20.

  ➢ Renal: dialysis dependent.

  ➢ Neurologic: severe, irreversible neurologic event/condition with high expected mortality.

*Forced expiratory volume in 1 second, a measure of lung function.
**Model of end-stage liver disease.

The MQS is a concept originating in military triage that informs critical care resource commitments. A critically ill casualty may be consuming resources that could save several other casualties, and his/her resource allocation may be reduced or withdrawn by establishing a ceiling on resource expenditure.[23] Both the MQS and exclusion criteria (Table 2-3) use the SOFA score to identify casualties likely to benefit from treatment, as well as those who are too sick to recover despite care. The SOFA score (Table 2-4) uses clinical and laboratory variables (arterial oxygen pressure [PaO_2], bilirubin, creatinine) to predict outcome by

TABLE 2-4 Sequential Organ Failure Assessment (SOFA) Score[24]

Variable	0	1	2	3	4
PaO_2/FiO_2, mm Hg	>400	≤400	≤300	≤200	≤100
Platelets, × 10^3/μL (× 10^6/L)	>150 (>150)	≤150 (≤150)	≤100 (≤100)	≤50 (≤50)	≤20 (≤20)
Bilirubin, mg/dL (μmol/L)	<1.2 (<20)	1.2–1.9 (20–32)	2.0–5.9 (33–100)	6.0–11.9 (101–203)	>12 (>203)
Hypotension	None	MABP <70 mm Hg	Dopamine ≤5	Dopamine >5, Epi ≤0.1, Norepi ≤0.1	Dopamine >15, Epi >0.1, Norepi >0.1
Glasgow Coma Scale score	15	13–14	10–12	6–9	<6
Creatinine, mg/dL (μmol/L)	<1.2 (<106)	1.2–1.9 (106–168)	2.0–3.4 (169–300)	3.5–4.9 (301–433)	>5 (>434)

Score is calculated by adding the value for each variable. MABP, mean arterial blood pressure; Epi, epinephrine; Norepi, norepinephrine. Dopamine, epinephrine, and norepinephrine values are in micrograms per kilogram per minute; SI units are given in parentheses.

TABLE 2-5 Critical Care Triage Tool (Initial Assessment)[23]

Triage Color Code	Criteria	Action/Priority
Blue	➤ Exclusion criteria met or ➤ SOFA score >11*	➤ Medical management ➤ Provide palliative care as needed ➤ Discharge from critical care
Red	➤ SOFA score ≤7 or ➤ Single organ failure	Highest priority
Yellow	SOFA score 8 to 11	Intermediate priority
Green	No significant organ failure	➤ Defer or discharge ➤ Reassess as needed

*If an exclusion criterion is met or the SOFA score exceeds 11 at any time between the initial assessment and 48 hours, change triage code to blue and proceed as indicated.

TABLE 2-6 Exclusion Criteria Prompting Reallocation of Lifesaving Interventions[26]

Sequential Organ Failure Assessment (SOFA) score criteria: casualties excluded from critical care if risk of hospital mortality >80%	Severe, chronic disease with short life expectancy

A. SOFA >15
B. SOFA >5 for >5 d, and with flat or rising trend
C. >6 organ failures
	A. Severe trauma
	B. Severe burns on patient with any two of the following:
	  i. Age >60 y
	  ii. >40% of total body surface area affected
	  iii. Inhalational injury
	C. Cardiac arrest
	  i. Unwitnessed cardiac arrest
	  ii. Witnessed cardiac arrest, not responsive to electrical therapy (defibrillation or pacing)
	  iii. Recurrent cardiac arrest
	D. Severe baseline cognitive impairment
	E. Advanced untreatable neuromuscular disease
	F. Metastatic malignant disease
	G. Advanced and irreversible neurologic event or condition
	H. End-stage organ failure
	I. Age >85 yr
	J. Elective palliative surgery

assessing the degree of organ system dysfunction and is one of the least complex and most predictive available metrics for prognosis prediction in critical care. It was developed to assist in determining the prognosis of a critically ill patient.[24]

During a large-scale disaster or public health emergency, scores such as SOFA can provide a means of objective prioritization of casualties when resources are overwhelmed and there is no adequate alternate measure. There are a number of physiologic scores from which to choose, but most of them require many additional laboratory values, are intended for use only at intensive care unit admission, may need 24 hours of information to be most predictive, and are not validated for longitudinal measurements of change that predict outcome. The disadvantages of SOFA include variables not designed for all populations (eg, Glasgow Coma Scale, creatinine), other variables that are modifiable by clinician actions without necessarily improving survival (eg, PaO_2/fraction of inspired oxygen [FiO_2]), lack of validation for pediatric populations, and uncertainty about cutoffs. In a large-scale disaster, many casualties may cluster around the same score, complicating further decisions.[25]

The MQS (Table 2-5) applies to initial casualty assessment for critical care.[21] Another issue is the reallocation of critical care resources, based on subsequent casualty response. Suggested criteria for such reallocation, listed in Table 2-6, are easier to discuss in the abstract than to apply in the real situation.[26]

2.6.5   Pediatric Considerations in Population-Based Triage

Population-based triage must make special provision not only for the pediatric population—especially infants and young children—but also for their families. Pediatric population-based triage must become a fully integrated component of public health and medical service disaster planning at all response levels—the involved community, the disaster scene, receiving hospitals, and the community and regional HEOC. Specifically, there should be a focus on the need to preserve family integrity whenever feasible, and to provide mechanisms for tracking pediatric patients and timely reunification of families whenever family integrity is impossible to maintain.[27]

This is fully analogous to the model that has long been promulgated by experts in emergency medical services for children, entitled *Prevention, Access, Life Support, and Specialized Care* (PALS), which facilitates involvement of pediatric experts throughout every phase of emergency preparedness and disaster management, while promoting a family-centered approach throughout the entire range of emergency care.[27]

2.7   INTEGRATION OF MASS CASUALTY AND POPULATION-BASED TRIAGE

While conceptually it is easy to consider mass casualty triage and population-based triage separately, in reality a large-scale disaster may require both forms of triage. For example, a large earthquake can damage a community's basic

TABLE 2-7 Integrated Mass Casualty and Population-Based Triage[21]

First-order triage management occurs at the community level to reduce disaster risks and define appropriate standards of care for the affected population.

Second-order triage management occurs at the prehospital/staging facility level to identify and care for casualties.

Third-order triage management occurs at hospitals and other receiving facilities to optimize opportunities for casualty survival within the constraints of available resources and procedures.

Fourth-order triage management occurs at the regional/state level to provide system-wide oversight and resource support for public health response efforts.

infrastructure, thus requiring population-based triage, while at the same time causing a significant building collapse, thus necessitating mass casualty triage at that scene. An emerging paradigm has been proposed for triage in a disaster of such a large magnitude. It takes a broader view of population-based triage management through a multi-tiered process that incrementally addresses mass care decision making under significant resource constraints and defines four orders of engagement within the health care system (Table 2-7).[21]

2.8 SUMMARY

Triage is the sorting of casualties by the seriousness of their condition and by the likelihood of their survival. It is used when health care needs exceed the immediately available resources. It is one of the most important tools of disaster health care response. The objective is to do the greatest good for the greatest number of possible survivors, when limited resources mean that not all casualties will be able to receive full medical care. Decisions made during triage will have an impact on the health outcomes of all affected individuals. Mass casualty triage rapidly categorizes casualties on the basis of their need for immediate medical attention. SALT triage is a simple method that rapidly sorts and assesses casualties for life-saving interventions, treatment, and transport. Responders and medical facility receivers should become familiar with the triage system used by their organization or agency and work to standardize the systems used across all components of the disaster response system in their community.

When an event results in widespread casualties and a community of individuals who are at risk for injury or illness, population-based triage should be considered. This involves not only obtaining care for the sick and injured but also protecting those who are not sick or injured. This includes region-wide risk communication and mitigation efforts, as well as transparent and fair resource allocation.

While mass casualty and population-based triage are taught as two distinct skills, in a large-scale catastrophic event, both may be required.

REFERENCES

1. Subbarao I, Lyznicki J, Hsu E, et.al. A consensus-based educational framework and competency set for the discipline of disaster medicine and public health preparedness. *Disaster Med Public Health Prep.* 2008:2;57–68.

2. Lerner EB, O'Connor RE, Schwartz R, et al. Blast-related injuries from terrorism: an international perspective. *Prehosp Emerg Care.* 2007;11(2):137–153.

3. Lerner EB, Schwartz RB, Coule PL, et al. Mass casualty triage: an evaluation of the data and development of a proposed national guideline. *Disaster Med Public Health Prep.* 2008;2(suppl 1):S25–S34.

4. Lerner EB, Schwartz RB, Coule PL, Pirrallo RG. Use of SALT triage in a simulated mass-casualty incident. *Prehosp Emerg Care.* 2010;14(1):21–25.

5. Benson M, Koenig K, Schultz C. Disaster triage: START, then SAVE—a new method of dynamic triage for victims of a catastrophic earthquake. *Prehosp Disaster Med.* 1996;11:117–124.

6. Kerby JD, MacLennan PA, Burton JN, McGwin G Jr, Rue LW III. Agreement between prehospital and emergency department Glasgow Coma Scores. *J Trauma.* 2007;63(5):1026–1031.

7. Romig L. The JumpSTART Pediatric MCI Triage Tool. January 2, 2008. http://www.jumpstart-triage.com/JumpSTART_and_MCI_Triage.php. Accessed February 10, 2008.

8. Nocera A, Garner A. An Australian mass casualty incident triage system for the future based upon triage mistakes of the past: the Homebush Triage Standard. *Aust N Z J Surg.* 1999;69(8):603–608.

9. Wiseman DB, Ellenbogen R, Shaffrey CI. Triage for the neurosurgeon. *Neurosurg Focus.* 2002;12(3):E5.

10. Hodgetts T, Hall J, Maconochie I, Smart C. Paediatric triage tape. *Prehosp Immediate Care.* 1998;2:155–159.

11. Navin D, Sacco W, Waddell R. Operational Comparison of the Simple Triage and Rapid Treatment Method and the Sacco Triage Method in Mass Casualty Exercises. J Trauma. 2010;69:215–222.

12. Hines S, Payne A, Edmondson J, Heightman AJ. Bombs under London: the EMS response plan that worked. *JEMS.* 2005;30(8):58–60, 62, 64–67.

13. Garner A, Nocera A. "Sieve," "sort" or START. *Emerg Med (Fremantle).* 2001;13(4):477.

14. Nocera A, Garner A. Australian disaster triage: a colour maze in the Tower of Babel. *Aust N Z J Surg.* 1999;69(8):598–602.

15. Frykberg E. Triage: principles and practice. *Scand J Surg.* 2005;94(4):272–278.

16. Hirschberg A, Scott B, Granchi T, et al. How does casualty load affect trauma care in urban bombing incidents? A quantitative analysis. *J Trauma.* 2005;58(4):686–693.

17. Armstrong J, Hammond J, Hirshberg A, Frykberg E. Is overtriage associated with increased mortality? The evidence says "yes." *Disaster Med Public Health Prep.* 2008;2(1):4–5.

18. Cone DC, Serra J, Burns K, MacMillan DS, Kurland L, Van Gelder C. Pilot test of the SALT mass casualty triage system. *Prehosp Emerg Care*. 2009;13(4):536–540.

19. Burkle FM Jr. Population-based triage management in response to surge-capacity requirements during a large-scale bioevent disaster. *Acad Emerg Med*. 2006;13(11):1118–1129.

20. World Health Organization. *Pandemic Influenza Preparedness and Response: A WHO Guidance Document*. Geneva, Switzerland: WHO; 2009. http://www.who.int/csr/disease/influenza/PIPGuidance09.pdf. Accessed May 19, 2010.

21. Bostick N, Subbarao I, Burkle F, et al. Disaster triage systems for large-scale catastrophic events. *Disaster Med Public Health Prep*. 2008;2(suppl 1):S35–S39.

22. Powell T, Christ KC, Birkhead GS. Allocation of ventilators in a public health disaster. *Disaster Med Public Health Prep*. 2008;2:20–26.

23. Christian M, Hawryluck L, Wax R, et al. Development of a triage protocol for critical care during an influenza pandemic. *CMAJ*. 2006;175(11):1377–1381.

24. Ferreria FL, Bota DP, Bross A, et al. Serial evaluation of the SOFA score to predict outcome in critically ill patients. *JAMA*. 2001;286(14):1754–1758.

25. Hick J, Rubinson L, O'Laughlin D, Clinical review: allocating ventilators during large-scale disasters—problems, planning, and process. *Crit Care*. 2007;11(3):217–225.

26. Devereaux A, Christian MD, Dichter JR, Geiling JA, Rubinson L. Summary of suggestions from the Task Force for Mass Critical Care Summit, January 26–27, 2007. *Chest*. 2008;133(suppl):1S–7S.

27. Foltin G, Tunik M, Treiber M, Cooper A, eds. *Pediatric Disaster Preparedness: A Resource for Planning, Management, and Provision of Out-Of-Hospital Emergency Care*. Washington, DC: EMSC National Resource Center; 2008.

CHAPTER THREE

Health System Surge Capacity for Disasters and Public Health Emergencies

John H. Armstrong, MD

Italo Subbarao, DO, MBA

Jim Lyznicki, MS, MPH

Arthur Cooper, MD, MS

Eric Frykberg, MD

3.1 PURPOSE

This chapter provides a comprehensive all-hazards framework for establishing health system surge capacity and surge capability to meet the needs of adult and pediatric populations in disasters and public health emergencies. Particular focus is placed on surge issues in health care facilities.

3.2 LEARNING OBJECTIVES

After completing this chapter, readers will be able to:

➤ Describe an all-hazards taxonomy for *surge capacity* and *surge capability* in the context of preparedness and response to disasters and public health emergencies.

➤ List four primary support elements that contribute to the efficiency of surge capacity and capability.

➤ Delineate a tiered management system for integrating medical and health resources during large-scale emergencies.

➤ Discuss strategies for providing contingency and crisis surge capacity for health care facilities.

➤ Explain the purpose of exercises and drills for all-hazards preparation and planning for disasters and public health emergencies.

3.3   DISASTER MEDICINE AND PUBLIC HEALTH PREPAREDNESS COMPETENCIES ADDRESSED[1]

➤ Explain the purpose of disaster exercises and drills in regional, community, and institutional disaster preparation and planning. (1.1.4)

➤ Conduct hazard vulnerability assessments for your office practice, community, or institution. (1.1.5)

➤ Delineate your function and describe other job functions in institutional, community, and regional disaster response systems to ensure unified command and scalable response to a disaster or public health emergency. (3.1.2)

➤ Characterize institutional, community, and regional surge capacity assets in the public and private health response sectors, and the extent of their potential assistance in a disaster or public health emergency. (3.3.2)

➤ Develop and evaluate policies, plans, and strategies for predicting and providing surge capacity of institutional, community, and regional health systems for the management of mass casualties in a disaster or public health emergency. (3.3.3)

3.4   INTRODUCTION

Disasters and public health emergencies are scalable events. As such, health facilities and community health systems must have appropriate all-hazard strategies to scale capacity as needed for the demand of individual casualties and populations affected by such events. This involves much more than the usual patient care resources of facilities and systems. The ability to expand personnel, facility space, and equipment/supply resources to meet the added demands of casualty loads and populations far above normal is essential for a health system and community to achieve a successful response.

The 2009–2010 H1N1 influenza pandemic underscored the relevance of preparation for a public health emergency in which hundreds to thousands of people suddenly seek medical care. As this occurs over hours, days, or weeks, the overwhelming surge on the health care system could dramatically strain medical resources and compromise the ability of health care professionals to adhere to routine treatment procedures and conventional standards of care. Over the past few years, in anticipation of a severe pandemic of H5N1 ("bird flu") and other public health emergencies (eg, bioterrorism), many states and health care institutions have been developing pandemic and other emergency preparedness plans to enhance the ability of the health care system to respond to public health emergencies and mass casualty events.

Beyond pandemics, nations face the possibility of many other public health emergencies and disasters that could severely strain medical resources. For example, the detonation of an improvised nuclear device in a large city would cause massive numbers of injured and dead. Similarly, disasters caused by terrorism or by nature, such as wildfires, floods, earthquakes, and hurricanes, have the potential to overwhelm medical and public health systems. The effects of the mismatch between health needs and resources after a major disaster can be devastating, as shown by the well-chronicled events in the United States that followed Hurricane Katrina.[2,3]

From a community perspective, the mobilization and expansion of resources must be coordinated across clinical care, public health, and emergency management systems. Further, resource expansion must be integrated with strict management of public communications to minimize population anxiety, direct casualty flow to available resources, and reduce overall demand on those resources.

3.5 DEFINING SURGE CAPACITY AND CAPABILITY

There is no singular accepted definition for health system or health facility surge capacity and surge capability. The most commonly used definition of surge capacity in disaster response is the ability to accommodate a sudden, unexpected increase in casualty volume that exceeds the usual capacity of the health care system or facility.[4] Surge capacity generates space and resources. On the other hand, surge capability is the actual availability of services (personnel skills combined with resources) to meet specific types of casualty needs. Stated another way, surge *capacity* refers to resource *availability*, surge *capability* to resource *operability*.

Surge capacity can be measured by numbers of facilities *and* equipped space within these facilities, such as beds, imaging units, and operating rooms that could be operational for a sudden, overwhelming need. Surge capacity can be more readily quantified as the number of additional beds (US national goals are 20% bed augmentation for acute care services, 300% for critical care services)[5] and the number of casualties who can be accommodated within a facility (not every casualty needs a bed).[6] These metrics have tended to dominate planning. While effective surge capacity rapidly *accommodates* a large number of casualties from a defined mass-casualty event or pandemic, the space does not equate to care. It is what can be done in that space that ultimately matters more.

Surge capacity occurs on a continuum with three distinct phases[4,7]:

1. *Conventional phase.* Traditional and normal patient care facilities and staff meet normal goals in providing care, ie, the status quo.

2. *Contingency phase.* Minor adaptations are made that may have minor consequences for standards of care, but adaptations are not enough to result in significant changes to routine standards of care.

3. *Crisis phase.* The event causes a fundamental, systematic change in the health care system, and standards of care are significantly altered in this context.

Surge capability combines capacity with what can be done for the casualties. Surge capability is measured as the number of casualties who can receive specific services given available personnel skills and resources (ie, number of ventilated patients given available ventilators, ventilator-proficient physicians and nurses, respiratory therapists, and monitored settings). A more integrated approach defines surge capability as the number of critical casualties arriving per hour without compromising the level of care of those casualties (at or above 90% of optimal care standards). As the arrival rate of critical casualties increases, the care capability falls along the slope of a sigmoid curve (Figure 3-1).[8] The critical population includes not only the critical casualties from the event, but also critically-ill patients with demands unrelated to the disaster, such as myocardial infarction, stroke, labor, and acute illness.

Four interdependent factors contribute to effective surge response: systems and infrastructure, space, staff, and supplies. Systems and infrastructure include the incident command framework, coordinated internal and external communications, and continuity of operations; without these, the other variables cannot be fully managed.[4]

FIGURE 3-1
Critical Casualty Load vs
Mean Global Level of Care

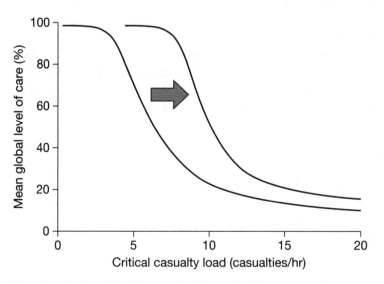

Adapted from Hirshberg.[8] Note that an effective disaster plan shifts the curve to the right by mobilizing surge capability.

3.6 A SURGE CAPACITY FRAMEWORK FOR HEALTH CARE FACILITIES

In a large-scale disaster or public health emergency, the influx of casualties creates a spectrum of supply and demand challenges for health care facilities. To adapt to changing resources (space, clinical and public health staff, and key supplies), an effective surge capacity plan must reflect the continuum of needs that vary according to the magnitude of the event. As the imbalance increases between resource availability and demand, a health care facility must move across the phases of surge capacity, first maximizing conventional capacity, then generating contingency capacity, and finally mobilizing crisis capacity. Similar events may result in conventional care at a major urban trauma center, while requiring crisis care at a smaller facility.[4]

Conventional, Contingency, and Crisis Capacity[4]

Conventional capacity—spaces, staff, and supplies used in daily practice within the institution. These can be used during a major mass casualty incident that triggers activation of the facility emergency operations plan.

Contingency capacity—spaces, staff, and supplies not used in daily practice, yet *functionally equivalent* to usual practice. These may be used temporarily during a major mass casualty incident and on a more sustained basis during a disaster (when the demands of the incident exceed community resources).

Crisis capacity—adaptive spaces, staff, and supplies outside usual standards of care, yet sufficient (ie, the best possible care to casualties given the circumstances and resources available) in the setting of a catastrophic disaster. Crisis capacity activation constitutes a *significant* adjustment to provision of care.

Concurrent with the transition along a surge capacity continuum is the realization that the standard of care will shift. This shift results from the growing scarcity of personnel and material resources needed to treat, transport, and provide casualty care. Goals for the health care facility are twofold: cope with the existing situation by maximizing the greatest good for the greatest number of casualties presenting to the facility, while working to return to conventional care by transferring casualties out of the area and drawing on health system resources. In moving to crisis capacity, the health care facility has the responsibility to evacuate casualties and staff as resources and the situation permit.

In a catastrophic event, a number of strategies can be implemented along the care continuum to accommodate changes in standards of care. These involve steps to substitute, conserve, adapt, and reuse critical resources, and ways that staff can be reassigned to deliver care. All of these steps should be attempted prior to the reallocation of critical resources in short supply. Every attempt must be made to maximize the greatest good for the population of casualties.[9]

3.6.1   Casualty Space Strategies

Adequate physical space and appropriate physical structures are often under-estimated needs in a disaster. Triage, treatment (including critical care), transportation staging, and discharge holding areas need to be initiated rapidly through transformation of existing nonclinical areas, such as lobby areas, gymnasiums, or conference rooms. Additional considerations include space and logistics for staff, family, and media.

Obtaining physical space in many health care facilities is a challenge, as most function near full capacity and have little available reserve space. Most facilities do not hold patients who are otherwise ready for discharge, and most ICU patients remain there until they no longer need intensive care.

Conventional patient space strategies include using all available staffed beds, mobilizing staff so that any unstaffed beds can be used, adding beds to usual patient rooms, canceling elective surgeries, using observation beds for inpatient care, activating surge discharge plans (reverse triage), and canceling onsite clinic appointments to free up clinic space and staff.[4]

Reverse Triage to Enhance Hospital Surge Capacity

Reverse triage is the process of rapidly identifying patients who can be safely discharged home, moved to an alternate care site, or transferred to a skilled nursing facility. Plans should provide guidance to expedite discharge to safe dispositions. Pre-disaster liaison with home health care agencies and long-term care facilities is crucial to the success of these early discharges. There is substantial variation between institutions in the percentage of patients appropriate for surge discharge; although 20% is a commonly used figure, this is likely exaggerated. It is important for hospitals to evaluate these measurements on the basis of institutional exercises.[10]

Contingency patient space strategies include providing inpatient care in areas that have appropriate medical infrastructure but are not typically used for this purpose, or providing a higher level of care than usual on inpatient units. This includes using post-anesthesia/pre-induction areas (particularly recovery beds in outpatient surgery and procedure areas) and procedural suites (endoscopy units, interventional cardiology or radiology) for inpatient care, as well as step-down, observation, or floor beds for higher levels of care. These sites should be used to manage casualty influx, with subsequent casualty movement to other areas or facilities as they become available.[4]

Crisis patient space strategies involve provision of inpatient care in areas that are not usually used for patient care. These include facility "flat space" areas such as conference rooms, hallways, and physical therapy gyms that can be readily outfitted with fixed or deployable systems for electrical power, oxygen supply, and vacuum suction; adjacent flat space areas, such as those appropriate for tenting; adjacent physician office space; and other offsite locations for non-ambulatory care.[4]

Table 3-1 provides an overview of possibilities for space, and Table 3-2 gives an example of surge capacity by bed count.

TABLE 3-1 Hospital Space Creation Strategies for a Major Incident[4]

	Time (hours)			
	0 to 2	**2 to 4**	**4 to 12**	**12 to 24**
Conventional	Fill available staffed beds; cancel elective procedures/surgeries and on-site clinics; use "in-place" bed additions—day beds in patient rooms converted to patient beds; begin reverse triage	Provide staff for unstaffed but available beds; add in-storage beds to usual patients' rooms; surge discharge opens beds; patients moved to pre-identified holding area	Add additional beds to existing patient rooms	Cancelation of elective cases begins to have impact, but does not open new beds
Contingency	Clear patients from pre-induction and procedure areas and fill available beds	Pre-induction and procedural areas fully available; transfer patients from higher-acuity care areas to lower-acuity care areas according to facility plan (from ICU to step down)	Assessment of situation—consider mechanisms to return to conventional care and request necessary resources	Initiate processes (internal or external transfers) to return to conventional care if possible
Crisis	Place patients in hallways or lobby areas on prestaged cots	Set up planned facility areas for austere impatient care	Mobilize resources for alternate care sites	Begin patient transfer to alternate care sites
Evacuation*	Evaluate facility impact and options for patient transfer	Arrange local/interregional patient transfers to return to at least contingency care operations and/or request necessary resources	Begin local and regional patient transfers	Begin federally facilitated (National Disaster Medical System) patient transfer

* If evacuation of patients is not possible, then activate crisis standards of care plan.

TABLE 3-2 Sample Calculation of Surge Capacity Space in a 400-bed Hospital[4]

	Calculation	**Notes**
a. Operating beds—average daily census	400 - 380 = 20	Represents average day; system monitoring will allow accurate forecasting at the time of an event; variability likely to be -20 to +20

(Continued)

TABLE 3-2 *(Continued)*

	Calculation	Notes
b. Usual surge discharge capability	400 x 0.15 = 60	Established by exercises (institution specific); here 15% could be discharged safely
c. Available beds to convert single to double rooms	20	Available beds in storage or already in rooms
Conventional capacity total	a + b + c = 100	
d. Procedure and post-anesthesia care beds	30	Enhanced critical care capability
Contingency capacity total	a + b + c + d = 130	

3.6.2 Staffing Strategies

Early mobilization of appropriately trained staff to fulfill needs imposed by disasters enhances effective response. A staff staging area or labor pool helps to centralize and organize staff deployment. A system must be in place to manage staff (both volunteer and regular) in order to use them efficiently and avoid diverting resources to activities such as ad hoc verification of credentials. Additional staff may be available from local facilities with preexisting staff sharing agreements. Prior agreements that detail shared staff compensation, liability coverage, and workers' compensation will improve staff sharing. Staff relief must be monitored continuously to adjust the response to the event as it evolves over time.

Conventional staffing strategies involve distribution of staff who are credentialed and privileged at the institution before the event. Staff at an institution may be assigned in their usual area or assigned to other patient areas, yet remain conventional staff as long as their skill sets are consistent with the duties assigned. Further, personnel duties following a disaster may be less differentiated than usual daily duties, ie, transformation from specialty to general care providers.

Fortunately, few hospitals experience staffing shortages during disasters, although in smaller facilities or with an event that poses a threat to responders, staff may be inadequate to meet casualty needs. In such situations, work practices must be modified to allow existing staff to expand capability for casualty care activities and may include reduction in care documentation, closing of non-essential departments to support others, and relaxation of nurse-to-patient ratios. Certain statutes and regulations may require modification in these instances and will require assistance from government agencies.[4]

Contingency staffing strategies include augmentation of existing staff with outside personnel who have a similar level of credentials and are pre-privileged or able to be privileged quickly (eg, partner hospital, Medical Reserve Corps, and state or federal medical response teams). Contingency staffing also involves provider "extension" into noncritical responsibilities. Use of contingency staff should prompt consideration of the risk-benefit ratio from importing staff to provide casualty care, compared to casualty evacuation to another facility with better resources.[4]

Staffing and Workforce Protection

The recent H1N1 pandemic and severe acute respiratory syndrome (SARS) experiences have consistently identified health care workers as an at-risk group for absenteeism (greater than 50%) due to concerns about clinical exposure.[11] Issues of greatest concern include:

➤ Family safety.

➤ Personal safety.

➤ Dependent child care.

➤ Transportation.

➤ Dependent adult care.

Pet care must also be considered. Key factors that positively influenced willingness of health care workers to work included the provision of medications (ie, antivirals) and personal protective equipment (ie, N-95 respirators) to the workers and their families. Worker protection issues are discussed further in Chapter 6.

Crisis staffing strategies used for catastrophic incidents that overwhelm hospital systems require the use of staff to perform clinical duties beyond what they usually perform, in order to provide the "greatest good for the greatest number of patients." Staff performance of clinical care that is above the scope of their usual responsibilities or training should be considered crisis care unless it carries a negligible risk to the casualty (Table 3-3). The use of crisis staffing should be part of a systematic process to concentrate all institutional resources on critical casualty care while obtaining additional qualified staff and initiating transfers to other facilities with higher casualty care capacity.[4]

TABLE 3-3 Sources and Responsibilities for Disaster Hospital Staffing[4]

	Source of Staff	**Possible Responsibilities**
Conventional	Facility staff providing care within usual scope, though location may be atypical	Staff surgeon assessing casualties in emergency department or providing care in postanesthesia area

(Continued)

TABLE 3-3 *(Continued)*

	Source of Staff	Possible Responsibilities
Contingency	Comparably trained and privileged staff from: ➤ Partner hospital (with a preexisting mutual aid agreement or within a health system). ➤ Hospital staff from local Medical Reserve Corp. ➤ Non-partner region/state hospital staff, interstate/federal personnel.	Intensive care nurses shared from partner hospital Burn nurses brought in from federal teams Critical care nurses provide direction to noncritical care nurses, rather than providing primary nursing care Workforce extension through reduction in administrative and noncritical/non-medical tasks
Crisis	Staff extending beyond assigned duties: ➤ Other hospital staff (not credentialed or privileged for these duties). ➤ Outside hospital staff (not usually credentialed or privileged for these duties). ➤ Partner outpatient clinic staff (same health system or with mutual agreement). ➤ Outpatient clinic staff from local Medical Reserve Corps. ➤ Licensed volunteer health care providers (must be credentialed by health care facility per their emergency credentialing/privileging standard). ➤ Medical reserve corps staff not currently licensed but with relevant clinical skills (retired physician or nurse, professional student). Lay volunteers	Ear, nose, and throat surgeon provides postoperative care for trauma patients Outpatient family physician from affiliated health care system provides inpatient care Lay volunteers assist with basic patient hygiene and nonmedical aspects of care and monitoring Retired surgeon provides postoperative care

3.6.3 Supply Strategies

In the business of daily health care delivery, surplus inventory and duplication of suppliers and services are discouraged, in favor of "just-in-time" inventory management. Consolidation of suppliers has also occurred, and suppliers maintain stocks sufficient only to meet anticipated orders. The supply chain is fragile, with little additional capacity.[4] Many hospitals rely on the same suppliers, further compounding resource shortfalls in a major disaster. If supplies are not available through existing channels, then mechanisms must be in place for the facility to obtain them from regional, state, or federal sources. This usually occurs via the local emergency management agency for the community in which the hospital is located.

An essential function within incident management is regular communication between operations and logistics to anticipate supply replacement needs in sufficient time to limit shortages (Table 3-4). A process of vendor-managed inventory by which private partners manage and store supplies for disasters has

TABLE 3-4 Options to Address Resource Shortages[4]

	Conventional	Contingency	Crisis
Prepare	Stockpile supplies		
Substitute	Equivalent medications (narcotic substitution)		
Conserve	Oxygen flow rates titrated to minimum required, discontinued for saturations >95%	Oxygen only for saturations <90%	Oxygen only for respiratory failure
Adapt		Anesthesia machine for mechanical ventilation	Bag valve manual ventilation
Reuse	Reuse cervical collars after surface disinfection	Reuse nasogastric tubes and ventilator circuits after appropriate disinfection	Reuse invasive lines after appropriate sterilization
Reallocate		Reallocate oxygen saturation and cardiac monitors only to those with critical illness	Reallocate ventilators to those with the best chance of a good outcome

been useful on the federal level as part of the Strategic National Stockpile. Local implementation of similar strategies can further improve the flow of supplies and equipment, lessening the burden on individual facilities or public partners to buy and store large caches of pharmaceuticals or supplies.

Conventional supply strategies should identify critical supplies that are needed in the first week and ensure sources of sufficient quantities of usual or equivalent materials. Stockpiling is an option and requires ongoing maintenance, as well as ready accessibility. Conventional supplies also may be obtained from other facilities and suppliers. These should be planned and their limitations noted (eg, distance, number of other hospitals relying on single supplier) before the event.[4]

Contingency supply strategies are required when usual supplies cannot be obtained, but an acceptable substitute can be used that accomplishes the objective without significant risk to casualties. Six options exist to mitigate or remediate supply shortages[4]:

➤ *Prepare:* stockpile necessary items or their equivalents before the event.

➤ *Conserve:* use less of a resource by lowering dosage or changing utilization practices (administer oxygen only for documented oxygen saturations < 90%).

➤ *Substitute:* use a clinically equivalent item (substitute benzodiazepine sedation for propofol).

➤ *Adapt:* use items or technologies to provide sufficient care (use of transport ventilators or anesthesia machines instead of regular ventilators).

➤ *Reuse:* after appropriate disinfection or sterilization, reuse supplies (eg, nasogastric tubes).

➤ *Reallocate:* remove therapy or a monitor from one patient to give to another with a higher chance of benefit or greater need (eg, reallocation of ventilators).

Crisis supply strategies require care processes that adapt to resource shortages so that the greatest good for the greatest number is achieved. Examples include bag-valve ventilation if no ventilators are available; providing oxygen only to casualties with oxygen saturations less than 90%; and reallocation of lifesaving therapies to casualties with better chances of a good outcome. The Strategic National Stockpile should be considered crisis supply. Some states also have medication and ventilator stockpiles, which should be determined in the planning process.

Strategic National Stockpile (SNS)[12]

The SNS is a national repository of antibiotics, chemical antidotes, antitoxins, life-support medications, intravenous administration supplies, airway supplies, and basic wound care supplies. This "storehouse" is designed to supplement local and state supplies in the event of a national emergency at any place and time within the extended United States (including territories). Push Packages are positioned in strategic and secure locations to enable deployment within 12 hours. SNS assets may be deployed, at the request of the governor of the affected state, the Secretary of Health and Human Services, or the director of the Centers for Disease Control and Prevention (CDC). These assets should not be considered available for the initial response.

3.7   PEDIATRIC SURGE CONSIDERATIONS

Children represent approximately 25% of the US population, yet use a smaller proportion of inpatient hospital services. Compared with available adult resources, there are fewer pediatric hospital beds, pediatric specialists, and providers with experience caring for critically ill and injured children. When a public health emergency affects all population subgroups equally, 25% of casualties will be pediatric. The resources required to meet the special needs of pediatric casualties can be considerable: the younger the patient, the more age specific the care needs.[13]

Pediatric hospitals represent only 5% of all US hospitals. The majority of emergency department visits for access to care are made to general hospitals that treat adult and pediatric patients. Few US emergency departments have all of the supplies deemed essential for managing pediatric patient emergencies, and only half of hospitals approach a complete inventory of essential pediatric supplies.[13]

Although children may be proportionately represented among the casualties of most natural disasters, the same is usually not true for technological disasters and human conflict, where children are typically underrepresented and overrepresented, respectively. Moreover, the clinical needs of pediatric populations may be magnified relative to adult populations as a result of anatomic differences, immature immune systems, and less developed abilities to recognize danger and seek protection. As many as one-third of all pediatric casualties who become ill or injured during a disaster require critical care in a pediatric intensive care unit, while the number of available pediatric critical care beds in any given region may be severely limited or distributed in a way that limits access to health care facilities near the disaster scene. Strategies for expanding regional pediatric critical care capabilities include[14]:

➤ Rapid discharge from the pediatric intensive care unit of current critical patients eligible for intermediate (step-down) level care.

➤ Rapid identification of arriving pediatric emergency department casualties who will not likely require admission to the pediatric intensive care unit.

➤ Expansion of pediatric intensive care unit capacity by adding additional fully staffed, equipped, and monitored beds to existing units.

➤ Expansion of pediatric intensive care unit capacity by deploying additional beds and staff in monitored environments (post-anesthesia care units, endoscopy units).

➤ Use of associated adult intensive care unit facilities and staff to care for older children and adolescents.

➤ Training of pediatric inpatient care providers, including hospitalists, in hospitals with and without pediatric intensive care units, to provide intermediate level (step-down) care to older children and adolescents.

➤ Prearranged system for inter-facility transport of pediatric casualties requiring critical care to nearby hospitals with underutilized pediatric intensive care units.

➤ Reallocation of resources to pediatric casualties based on the likelihood of better outcomes, according to preexisting guidelines that have been developed with community input.[15]

It bears emphasis that, in a disaster, casualties will not discriminate between adult and pediatric hospitals. All hospitals must have a basic readiness for casualties across demographics.

3.8 ADDITIONAL SURGE CONSIDERATIONS

Certain situations require specialized surge responses. Patients contaminated by radioactive materials from a radiologic dispersion device ("dirty bomb") may have combined injuries that require radiologic decontamination and injury management. Other specialized situations include highly infectious, burn, or chemical casualties. These situations may require assignment of staff with specific training relative to these hazards and specialized resources (eg, radiologic survey meters and personal protective equipment).

3.9 ALTERNATE CARE FACILITIES (SITES) IN SURGE CAPACITY

During large-scale disasters or pandemics, health care facilities will likely run out of space. Alternate areas will be needed for minimal casualties, families, the worried well, and mass volunteer providers. Possibilities include parking garages, grouped ambulances, schools, churches, malls, civic/community centers, and medical/dental professional offices. When considering possibilities, it is important to define availability (eg, students are in schools on weekdays) and expectations through memoranda of agreement. To be effective, alternate care sites should be defined before the event; trying to identify new space in the midst of the disaster is too late.[16] Emergency Medical Treatment and Labor Act (EMTALA) provisions hold for hospital-based alternate care sites (ie, on the hospital campus), but not for off-campus screening facilities or non-hospital alternate care sites.[17]

There is a distinction between *health care facility* surge capacity and *community* surge capacity: community surge capacity strategies focus on the creation of out-of-hospital solutions to the delivery of health care. This understanding has led to the emergence of the alternate care facility (ACF): a location for the delivery of medical care outside the acute hospital setting for casualties who, under normal circumstances, would be treated in a hospital. The ACF is also viewed as a site to provide event-specific management of unique considerations that arise in the context of catastrophic mass casualty events, including the delivery of long-term care; the distribution of vaccines or medical countermeasures; and the quarantine, cohorting, or sequestration of potentially infectious casualties with easily transmissible infectious disease.[18]

The selection of a facility for use as an ACF is an imprecise science and varies according to the nature of the event. Using a consensus process, a group of hospital engineers, facility personnel, and health care providers developed and refined a list of ACF infrastructure requirements based on initial work by the Department of Defense. These characteristics were then incorporated into an on-line matrix tool to assist in planning for ACF site selection, with each characteristic being assigned a relative weight from 0 to 5. Each facility under consideration is assigned a rank order based on the matrix calculation for ACF suitability, and a list of potential ACF options can be developed and maintained (see Appendix).[19]

Although the target population and scope of care at an ACF may be event-specific, some general guidelines are outlined in Table 3-5.

Depending on the extent of respiratory casualties, a key decision point in ACF selection for out-of-hospital care may be the ability to provide pulmonary support (oxygen, respiratory therapy, and/or mechanical ventilation). Nursing homes and long-term care facilities may be particularly useful, given their existing medical gas supplies. Otherwise, the logistics and expense of sustaining oxygen delivery systems in an ACF setting are very complex and very expensive.

Tentative sites are best identified in advance, and the mechanism of approval for use as an ACF should be investigated. Permission to use municipal buildings may be easier to obtain, along with memoranda of understanding to use existing staff members. Structures of opportunity vary depending on the proximity to, and nature of the event; space; existing facility occupancy; ease of movement of services into these facilities; and ease access when closed. Although ACF selection is usually a local function, state partners should be queried in the planning process about designation of potential shelters or ACFs at the state or regional level. If the ACF must supply ambulatory patient care, it may help to locate it

TABLE 3-5 Alternative Care Facility (ACF) Scope of Care[19]

Scope of Care	Objectives of ACF Implementation	Scenario Type	Facility Type
Delivery of ambulatory/ long-term care/special medical needs	Decompression of medi-cal shelters and emer-gency departments	All	ACF
Receiving site for hos-pital discharge patients (non–oxygen dependent)	Decompression of acute care hospital inpatient beds	All	ACF
Inpatient care for moderate-acuity (non–oxygen-dependent) patients	Alterative to acute care hospital inpatient beds	All	ACF
Sequestration/ cohort-ing of "exposed" patient population	Protection of acute care hospitals from exposure to potentially infectious patients	Pandemic influenza/ bioevent	Home/ACF
Delivery of palliative care	Alternative to acute care hospital inpatient beds	All	Home/ACF

near a shelter in order to support casualties with chronic medical needs in that shelter. ACF options include[19]:

➤ Aircraft hangers.

➤ Churches.

➤ Community/recreation centers.

➤ Convalescent care facilities.

➤ Fairgrounds.

➤ Government buildings.

➤ Hotels/motels.

➤ Malls.

➤ Military facilities and tents.

➤ National guard armories.

➤ Same-day surgery centers and clinics.

➤ Schools.

➤ Shuttered hospitals.

➤ Sports facilities and stadiums.

3.10 SURGE CAPACITY AND CAPABILITY MANAGEMENT SYSTEM

Integration of all medical and public health assets in the community is a necessary step toward increasing response capacity and capability. This requires that disparate local health and medical organizations plan collaboratively for a coordinated, community-wide emergency response. Health response organizations should expect to work together during an emergency, but do not necessarily share plans or have a commonly understood framework for coordination under conditions of urgency and uncertainty in a rapidly evolving incident. The preferred framework is one in which the established health care system (hospital administrators, emergency departments, physicians, nurses, emergency medical services, community health clinics, pharmacists, and other caregivers) works closely with the public health community (state and local departments of health and their partners) in explicit linkage with the local emergency management agency.

Public health organizations (federal, state, and local) have an important role in helping to ensure appropriate care for all ages and populations through health monitoring, disease surveillance, and laboratory sciences. Additionally, the public health system acts as the expert system for tracking, predicting, and developing response tactics to disease outbreaks or other health threats. The public health system has a role in communicating prevention strategies as well as information about self-care and shelter-in-place during a crisis. In an emergency, the public also may be advised to seek care or reassurance in alternate settings so that hospitals and emergency care facilities can focus resources on the critically injured who need them most.

The US Department of Health and Human Services (HHS) Medical Surge Capacity and Capability (MSCC) Management System describes a public health and medical response system, consistent with the National Incident Management System (NIMS), for the coordination and integration all appropriate response entities at government levels.[20] The NIMS establishes core concepts and organizational processes based on incident command principles to allow diverse disciplines from all levels of government and the private sector to work together in response to domestic hazards. NIMS compliance is required of all federal departments and agencies, as well as state, tribal, and jurisdictional organizations, that seek federal preparedness assistance.

The MSCC Management System is a tiered response management framework for integrating medical and public health resources during large-scale emergencies (Table 3-6; Figure 3-2). It describes a process for expanding the scale of response from the individual health care organization (tier 1) through the health care coalition (tier 2), to local (tier 3), state (tier 4), interstate (tier 5), and federal (tier 6) levels.[20] The MSCC Management System reflects the reality that disasters do not respect organizational boundaries and geographic borders.

TABLE 3-6 HHS MSCC Management System[20]

Tier	Level	Function
Tier 6	Federal response	Support to state and locals
Tier 5	Interstate regional coordination	Management coordination and mutual support
Tier 4	State response and coordination of intrastate jurisdictions	Management coordination and support to jurisdictions
Tier 3	Jurisdiction incident management	Medical incident command system (ICS) and emergency support—emergency operations center (EOC)
Tier 2	Health care "coalition"	Information sharing, cooperative planning, mutual aid
Tier 1	Health care asset management	Emergency management program + emergency operations plan using incident command

FIGURE 3-2

HHS Medical Surge Capacity
and Capability (MSCC)
Framework[20]

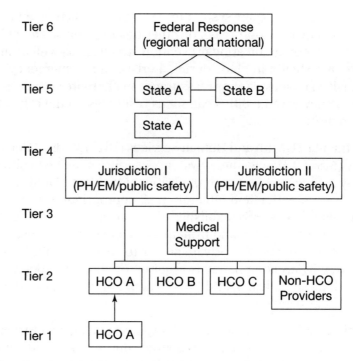

PH = public health; EM = emergency management; HCO = health care organization.

Tier 1: management of individual health care assets. A well-defined ICS to collect and process information, to develop incident plans, and to manage decisions is essential to maximize MSCC. Robust processes must be applicable both to traditional hospital participants and to other health care organizations that may provide patient care in an emergency, such as outpatient clinics, community health centers, urgent care centers, and private physician offices, among others. Each health care asset must have communication and information management processes to enable integration within the organization and with higher management tiers.[20]

Tier 2: management of a health care coalition. Coordination among local health care assets is critical to provide adequate and consistent care across an affected jurisdiction. The health care coalition provides central integration for information sharing and management coordination among health care assets, and it also establishes an effective and balanced approach to integrating medical assets into the jurisdiction's ICS (incident command system).

The concept of a health care coalition is an emerging model for community preparedness, planning, and response. The health care coalition is composed of health care facilities and other health and medical assets that form a single functional entity to maximize medical surge capacity and capability in a defined geographic area. It coordinates the mitigation, preparedness, response, and recovery actions of medical and health providers; facilitates mutual aid support; and serves as a unified platform for sharing medical input with jurisdictional authorities.[21]

Tier 3: local incident management. A jurisdiction's ICS integrates health care assets with other response disciplines to provide the structure and support needed to maximize MSCC. In certain events, the jurisdictional ICS promotes a unified incident command that allows multiple response entities, including public health and clinical, to assume significant management responsibility.[20]

Tier 4: management of state response. State governments participate in medical incident response across a range of capacities, depending on the specific event. The state may be the lead incident command authority; may provide support to incidents managed at the jurisdictional level (tier 3); or may coordinate multijurisdictional incident response. Common concepts are delineated to accomplish all of these missions, ensuring that the full range of state public health and medical resources is brought to bear to maximize MSCC.[20]

Tier 5: interstate regional management coordination. Effective mechanisms must be implemented to promote incident management coordination between affected states. This ensures consistency in regional response through coordinated incident planning, enhances information exchange between interstate jurisdictions, and maximizes MSCC through interstate mutual aid and other support. Tier 5 incorporates existing instruments, such as the Emergency Management Assistance Compact (EMAC, discussed in chapter 5.), and describes established incident command and mutual aid concepts to address these critical needs.[20]

Tier 6: federal support to state, tribal, and jurisdiction management. Effective management processes at the state (tier 4) and local (tier 3) levels facilitate the request, receipt, and integration of federal public health and clinical resources to maximize MSCC.[20]

The tiers of the MSCC Management System must be fully coordinated with each other and with the nonmedical incident response. The processes that promote this coordination and integration enable clinical care and public health to move beyond their traditional roles and become competent participants in large-scale medical incident management. The MSCC Management System provides an overarching model that can help to organize seemingly disparate public and private medical response assets. With its basis in ICS, the MSCC Management System helps to ensure that medical and public health organizations develop NIMS-consistent relationships, strategies, processes, and procedures, and become equal partners who are fully integrated into the emergency response community.

3.11 PLANNING AND PRACTICE FOR HEALTH SYSTEM SURGE CAPACITY

3.11.1 Hazard Vulnerability Analysis

All-hazards planning for surge capacity in disasters is stimulated by a hazard vulnerability analysis (HVA), a needs assessment that defines high-probability, high-risk events for which a healthcare system should be prepared. These potential events are then reviewed through the lens of existing readiness across events to define gaps that require attention and surge resources.[22] An HVA is straightforward (Table 3-7):

TABLE 3-7 Hazard Vulnerability Analysis

Event	Probability	Risk	Level of Preparation
Natural disasters			
Technological disasters			
Infectious disease outbreaks (foodborne, waterborne, pandemic)			
Terrorism			

➤ Make a list of possible events that could become disasters in the community across natural and human-caused (intentional or unintentional) events.

➤ Determine the probability (high, medium, low, rare) of, and risk from each potential event. For example, hurricanes in the US have a high probability of occurring from June through November each year along the Gulf Coast and causing casualties with loss of infrastructure.

➤ Assess the current level of preparedness and define the preparedness gap, which includes surge capacity and capability.

The HVA makes planning relevant to communities based on geography, industry, and demographics, including special needs populations. Planning based on the all-hazards model identifies common denominator issues across all scenarios and produces a higher level of preparedness than scenario-specific planning, which expands the universe of possibilities toward less likely events and leads to hit-or-miss results. Examining illness and injury distributions across mass casualty scenarios can help to identify a common set of surge elements that are necessary to provide care, irrespective of the nature of the disaster. Examples include respiratory support for the care of casualties with anthrax and botulism; management of multidimensional acute traumatic injuries; burns caused by nuclear events, industrial explosions, and highrise fires; decontamination for radioactive agents, anthrax spores, or nerve agents; and isolation requirements for multiple biologic agents and pandemic influenza.[22]

3.11.2 Practicing the Plan

Accreditation of healthcare organizations is one mechanism to reinforce the importance of hospital disaster preparedness. In the US, the Joint Commission (TJC) does this for hospitals through standard-setting and site surveys. TJC defines an *emergency* as an unexpected or sudden event that increases demand for care and disrupts the ability to provide care or the environment of care, whereas a *disaster* is a higher-order event by complexity, scope, or duration. Disaster threatens capabilities, which are bolstered by surge capabilities for care, safety, or security.[23]

In 2008, training for disasters was incorporated as a new element in TJC Environment of Care Emergency Management Standards, EC.4.18: "The organization establishes strategies for managing clinical and support activities during emergencies." Relevant emergency management (EM) standards include the following[23]:

➤ Participation of medical leaders in hazard vulnerability analysis (HVA) (EM.01.01.01).

➤ Establishment of response procedures for 96 hours (EM.02.01.01).

➤ Communication requirements including alternatives (EM.02.02.01).

➤ Family support plan for staff (EM.02.02.07).

➤ Surge, casualty tracking, and evacuation (EM.02.02.11).

➤ Privileges for volunteer providers, with oversight < 72 hours (EM.02.02.13).

➤ Two drills/exercises per year, excluding tabletops (EM.03.01.03). The drills should include an influx of simulated casualties and community participation.

Hospital disaster plans can be exercised in three ways. The first involves the desktop simulation exercise, often called a "tabletop exercise," using paper, verbal, or computer-based scenarios designed to improve staff coordination, communication, and decision making. Paper drills are often done to demonstrate "how response functions work" through communication in the Hospital Incident Command System (HICS).[24]

A second method, "functional exercise," evaluates the entire hospital response. Functional exercises usually involve the activation and simulated activity of all sections of the HICS and test the disaster plan in simulated field conditions.[24]

The third method, "field exercise drill," allows hospital staff to interact with each other, learn about their respective roles, gain experience working with the hospital and community plan, and understand what must be done under a realistic training environment. Drills often involve coordination of prehospital and hospital response personnel and take place in real time, as they test the mobilization, including the activation of the health component of the EOC (representatives of health care facilities, agencies, and organizations). Because disasters often cross political, geographic, functional, and jurisdictional boundaries, drills and training are most effective when carried out on a multi-organizational, multidisciplinary, and multi-jurisdictional basis. Evaluators observe the action, report on what went well and what did not, assess whether the goals and objectives were met, and report on how the participants performed. On the basis of the evaluation results, the hospital plan may be revised.[24] A list of resources for health care facility surge capacity planning is included in the Appendix.

3.12 SUMMARY

Surge capacity refers to the ability of health care facilities and systems to expand resources to care for casualties. *Surge capability* refers to the application of these expanded resources to the actual care of casualties. Establishing surge capacity to meet increased health-related needs in a disaster consists of four primary support elements: staff (human resources), space (facilities), supplies (stuff), and system (integrated infrastructure to mobilize and allocate resources). The availability of resources is limited by the routine needs of a community and by the economics and logistics involved in creating and maintaining excess capacity within normal community requirements for a mass casualty event. Casualty hospital bed availability becomes a critical factor, especially for those hospitals in proximity to the disaster scene.

In a large-scale disaster or public health emergency, hospital staff will have to deal with an influx of casualties who need or think they need prompt attention. This response can overwhelm health care facilities. Such overloading not only may exhaust resources at the facility but may shut it down altogether because of overcrowding or contamination. The challenge remains how to meet mass casualty demands while continuing to meet the needs of patients who are already receiving care in the facility before the event and the additional patients who may present in the coming hours with illness and injury unrelated to the event. Processes to obtain additional capacity during a disaster must be pre-established and flexible, with predetermined methods of activating these resources for different levels of response. Planning for surge requires forethought; surge as afterthought expands the disaster.

REFERENCES

1. Subbarao I, Lyznicki J, Hsu E, et.al. A consensus-based educational framework and competency set for the discipline of disaster medicine and public health preparedness. *Disaster Med Public Health Prep.* 2008;2:57–68.

2. Berggren R, Curiel T. After the storm—health care infrastructure in post-Katrina New Orleans. *N Engl J Med.* 2006;354:1549–1552.

3. Johnston C, Redlener I, eds. Hurricane Katrina, children, and pediatric heroes: hands-on stories by and of our colleagues helping families during the most costly natural disaster in U.S. history. *Pediatrics.* 2006;117:S355–S460.

4. Hick J, Barbera J, Kelen G. Refining surge capacity: conventional, contingency, and crisis capacity. *Disaster Med Public Health Prep.* 2009;3(suppl 1):S59–S67.

5. Rubinson L, Hick JL, Hanfling D, et al. Definitive care for the critically ill during a disaster: a framework for optimizing critical care surge capacity: from a Task Force for Mass Critical Care summit meeting, January 26–27, 2007, Chicago, IL. *Chest.* 2008;133(5 suppl):18S–31S.

6. National Center for Injury Prevention and Control. *In A Moment's Notice: Surge Capacity for Terrorist Bombings.* Atlanta, GA: Centers for Disease Control and Prevention; 2010. http://www.bt.cdc.gov/masscasualties/pdf/CDC_Surge-508.pdf.

7. Altevogt B, Stroud C, Nadig L, Hougan M. *Medical Surge Capacity: Workshop Summary, Institute of Medicine Forum on Medical and Public Health Preparedness for Catastrophic Events.* Washington, DC: National Academies Press; 2010.

8. Hirshberg A, Scott B, Granchi T, et.al. How Does Casualty Load Affect Trauma Care in Urban Bombing Incidents? A Quantitative Analysis. *J Trauma.* 2005;58:686–695.

9. Institute of Medicine. *Guidance for Establishing Crisis Standards of Care for Use in Disaster Situations: A Letter Report.* Washington, DC: National Academies Press; 2009.

10. Kelen G, McCarthy M, Kraus C, et al. Creation of surge capacity by early discharge of hospitalized patients at low risk for untoward events. *Disaster Med Public Health Preparedness.* 2009;3(supp 1):S10–S16.

11. Garrett A, Park Y, Redlener I, Mitigating absenteeism in hospital workers during a pandemic. *Disaster Med Public Health Preparedness.* 2009;3(suppl 2):S141–S147.

12. Centers for Disease Control and Prevention. Emergency preparedness and response: Strategic National Stockpile (SNS). http://www.bt.cdc.gov/stockpile/. Accessed July 30, 2010.

13. Allen G, Parrillo S, Will J, Mohr J. Principles of disaster planning for the pediatric population. *Prehosp Disaster Med.* 2007;22:537–540.

14. Centers for Bioterrorism Preparedness Planning Pediatric Task Force, New York City Department of Health and Mental Hygiene. *Pediatric Disaster Tool Kit: Hospital Guidelines for Pediatrics in Disasters.* 2nd ed. New York, NY: New York City Dept of Health and Mental Hygiene; 2006. http://www.nyc.gov/html/doh/html/bhpp/bhpp-focus-ped-toolkit.shtml. Accessed July 30, 2010.

15. Kanter R, Andrake J, Boeing N, et al. Developing consensus on appropriate standards of disaster care for children. *Disaster Med Public Health Prep.* 2009;3:27–32.

16. Peleg K, Kellermann A. Enhancing hospital surge capacity for mass casualty events. *JAMA.* 2009;302(5):565–567.

17. Roszak A, Jensen F, Wild R, et al. Implications of the Emergency Medical Treatment and Labor (EMTALA) during public health emergencies and on alternate sites of care. *Disaster Med Public Health Preparedness.* 2009;3(suppl 2):S172–S175.

18. Cantrill S, Pons P, Bonnett C, et al. *Disaster Alternate Care Facilities: Selection and Operation.* Prepared by Denver Health under contract 290-20-0600-020. AHRQ publication 09-0062. Rockville, MD: Agency for Healthcare Research and Quality; October 2009.

19. Phillips S, Knebel A, eds. *Mass Medical Care with Scarce Resources: A Community Planning Guide.* Prepared by Health Systems Research Inc, an Altarum company, under contract 290-04-0010. AHRQ publication 07-0001. Rockville, MD: Agency for Healthcare Research and Quality; 2007.

20. Barbera J, Macintyre A. *Medical Surge Capacity and Capability: A Management System for Integrating Medical and Health Resources During Large Scale Emergencies.* 2nd ed. Washington, DC: US Dept of Health and Human Services; September 2007.

21. Barbera J, Macintyre A. *Medical Surge Capacity and Capability: The Healthcare Coalition in Emergency Response and Recovery.* Washington, DC: US Dept of Health and Human Services; May 2009.

22. Kaiser Permanente Healthcare Continuity Management and Washington Hospital Center ER One Institute. Hospital Incident Command System Guidebook. California Emergency Medical Services Authority; 2006. http://www.emsa.ca.gov/HICS/files/Guidebook_Glossary.pdf. Accessed December 15, 2009.

23. The Joint Commission, Hospital Accreditation Standards 2010: Accreditation Policies, Standards, Elements of Performance, Scoring. Chicago: Joint Commission Resources, 2010.

24. Emergency Management Institute. IS-139 exercise design, March 2003. http://training.fema.gov/EMIWeb/IS/is139lst.asp. Accessed July 30, 2010.

APPENDIX

Selected Surge Capacity Planning Guides and Tools

Agency for Healthcare Research and Quality

Altered Standards of Care for Mass Casualty Events (events with potential to generate thousands of ill/injured/contaminated). Available at http://www .ahrq.gov/research/altstand/index.html.

Disaster Alternate Care Facilities: Report and Interactive Tools. Available at http://www.ahrq.gov/prep/acfselection/dacfrep.htm.

Emergency Preparedness Atlas: US Nursing Home and Hospital Facilities. Available at http://www.ahrq.gov/prep/nursinghomes/atlas.htm. Adjunct report on nursing home special needs and potential roles available at http://www.ahrq.gov/prep/nursinghomes/report.htm.

Emergency Preparedness Resource Inventory (EPRI): A Tool for Local, Regional, and State Planners. Available at http://www.ahrq.gov/research/ epri/index.html.

Hospital Surge Model (interactive web-based tool for estimating incident impact). Available at http://hospitalsurgemodel.ahrq.gov/.

Pediatric Hospital Surge Capacity in Public Health Emergencies. Available at http://www.ahrq.gov/prep/pedhospital/.

Providing Mass Medical Care with Scarce Resources: A Community Planning Guide. Available at http://www.ahrq.gov/research/mce/.

Rocky Mountain Regional Care Model for Bioterrorist Events: Locate Alternate Care Sites During an Emergency (surge planning tool). Available at http://www.ahrq.gov/research/altsites.htm. Web-based facility scoring matrix available at http://www.ahrq.gov/research/altsites/.

Reopening Shuttered Hospitals to Expand Surge Capacity. Available at http://www.ahrq.gov/research/shuttered/.

California Hospital Association

Healthcare surge planning resources. Available at http://www.calhospital prepare.org/.

Centers for Medicare and Medicaid Services

EMTALA requirements and options for hospitals in a disaster (includes EMTALA pandemic surge fact sheet. Available at http://www.tvfr.com/ safetytips/emer_prep/hospital/docs/CMS-hospital_surge_081409.pdf.

CHEST Journal

Definitive Care for the Critically Ill During a Disaster. Series of articles available at http://chestjournal.chestpubs.org/content/133/5_suppl.

Institute of Medicine

Medical Surge Capacity: Workshop Summary. Available at http://www.nap.edu/catalog.php?record_id=12798.

Guidance for Establishing Crisis Standards of Care for Use in Disaster Situations: A Letter Report. Available at http://www.nap.edu/catalog.php?record_id=12749.

New York City Department of Health and Mental Hygiene

Pediatric Disaster Tool Kit: Hospital Guidelines for Pediatrics in Disasters. Available at: http://www.nyc.gov/html/doh/html/bhpp/bhpp-focus-ped-toolkit.shtml.

The Joint Commission

Guide to Providing Safe Care in Surge Hospitals. Available at http://www.jointcommission.org/assets/1/18/surge_hospital.pdf.

US Department of Health and Human Services

FluSurge 2.0. Available at http://www.cdc.gov/flu/tools/flusurge/.

National Center for Injury Prevention and Control. *In a Moment's Notice: Surge Capacity for Terrorist Bombings*. Atlanta, GA: Centers for Disease Control and Prevention; 2010. Available at http://www.bt.cdc.gov/masscasualties/pdf/CDC_Surge-508.pdf.

Medical Surge Capacity and Capability: A Management System for Integrating Medical and Health Resources During Large Scale Emergencies, September 2007. Available at http://www.phe.gov/Preparedness/planning/mscc/handbook/Documents/mscc080626.pdf.

Medical Surge Capacity and Capability: The Healthcare Coalition in Emergency Response and Recovery, May 2009. Available at http://www.phe.gov/Preparedness/planning/mscc/Documents/mscctier2jan2010.pdf.

CHAPTER FOUR

Community Health Emergency Operations and Response

Italo Subbarao, DO, MBA

Jim Lyznicki, MS, MPH

Dennis Amundson, DO, MS

Arthur Cooper, MD, MS

Frederick M. Burkle, Jr., MD, MPH, DTM

4.1 PURPOSE

This chapter describes the core structure and functions associated with health emergency operations and response at the community level. It discusses the tripartite integration of the health care, emergency management, and public health systems into a coherent framework that provides situational awareness, surveillance, risk communication, mass care, mass prophylaxis, and mass fatality management.

4.2 LEARNING OBJECTIVES

After completing this chapter, readers will be able to:

➤ Discuss the function of the public health system and infrastructure in community disaster preparedness, response, and recovery.

➤ Summarize the key health components and functions of an Emergency Operations Center (EOC) in a disaster or public health emergency.

➤ Describe the purpose of public health surveillance in preparing for, responding to, and recovering from disasters and public health emergencies.

➤ Discuss public health interventions for the prevention and management of the full spectrum of injuries, illnesses, and disabilities in all affected ages and populations in a disaster or public health emergency.

➤ Discuss issues and challenges in communicating health risks to all affected ages and populations during a disaster or public health emergency.

➤ Apply federal and institutional guidelines and protocols to mitigate disease transmission in a pandemic event.

➤ Describe elements of effective mass fatality management in a disaster event or public health emergency that results in high mortality.

➤ Discuss the rationale for building community resilience for disasters and public health emergencies.

➤ Discuss the elements of the after-action report following a disaster or public health emergency.

4.3   DISASTER MEDICINE AND PUBLIC HEALTH PREPAREDNESS COMPETENCIES ADDRESSED[1]

➤ Summarize your regional, community, office, institutional, and personal/family disaster plans. (1.1.3)

➤ Explain the purpose and role of surveillance systems that can be used to detect and monitor a disaster or public health emergency. (2.1.4)

➤ Describe emergency communication and reporting systems and procedures for contacting family members, relatives, coworkers, and local authorities in a disaster or public health emergency. (2.2.1)

➤ Use emergency communications systems to report critical health information to appropriate authorities in a disaster or public health emergency. (2.2.3)

➤ Describe strategies for and barriers to communicating and disseminating health information to all ages and populations affected by a disaster or public health emergency. (2.3.1)

➤ Delineate cultural, ethnic, religious, linguistic, and health-related issues that need to be addressed in regional, community, and institutional emergency communication systems for all ages and populations affected by a disaster or public health emergency. (2.3.2)

➤ Characterize institutional, community, and regional surge capacity assets in the public and private health response sectors, and the extent of their potential assistance in a disaster or public health emergency. (3.3.2)

➤ Use federal and institutional guidelines and protocols to prevent the transmission of infectious agents in health care and community settings. (4.1.3)

➤ Describe psychological, emotional, cultural, religious, and forensic considerations for the management of mass fatalities in a disaster or public health emergency. (5.3.1)

➤ Explain the implications and specialized support services required for the management of mass fatalities from natural disasters, epidemics, and acts of terrorism (eg, involving conventional and nuclear explosives and/or release of biologic, chemical, and radiological agents). (5.3.2)

➤ Explain the significance of (and the need to collect and preserve) forensic evidence from living and deceased humans and animals at a disaster scene or receiving facility. (5.3.3)

➤ Apply knowledge and skills for the public health management of all ages, populations, and communities affected by natural disasters, industrial- or transportation-related catastrophes, epidemics, and acts of terrorism, in accordance with professional scope of practice. This includes active/passive surveillance, movement restriction, vector control, mass immunization and prophylaxis, rapid needs assessment, environmental monitoring, safety of food and water, and sanitation. (5.4.2)

➤ Demonstrate creative and flexible decision making in various contingency situations and risk scenarios, under crisis conditions and with limited situational awareness. (6.1.2)

➤ Explain mechanisms for providing post-event feedback and lessons learned to appropriate authorities (eg, through after-action reports) to improve regional, community, and institutional disaster response systems. (6.2.3)

4.4 HURRICANE KATRINA: A SIREN CALL FOR HEALTH EMERGENCY RESPONSE SYSTEMS

With the 2001 terrorist attacks by plane and mailed anthrax in the United States, nations became more focused on preparedness and response for mass casualty events. There was a realization that, in order to be effective, preparedness and response efforts had to be better coordinated, not only within the medical and public health sectors, but also with other public and private stakeholders, who are essential to providing information and service to affected populations (such as transportation, law enforcement, business, and the media). Countless programs were developed to better educate, train, and equip health care responders for terrorism and other mass casualty events. Officials and leaders met frequently, policies began to emerge, and there was a general feeling that progress was being made and that national health security had improved.

In 2005, the aftermath of Hurricane Katrina along the US Gulf Coast was a reality check.[2-5] In the midst of extensive human suffering and economic damage, illusions about the ability of the world's superpower to launch a systematic, integrated health response were shattered.[2-5] Health-related needs and issues surfaced at a magnitude not previously experienced by local and state health officials, and traditional response and recovery operations could not meet all of the resulting human needs, in either the short or long term. A diversity of special health concerns, language and cultural barriers, and social class realities were exposed.

Traditionally, disaster preparation has not focused on the needs of survivors with preexisting chronic medical conditions, or on the needs of children, the aged, the disabled, and the displaced, but rather on acute injuries, environmental exposures, and infectious diseases. In the United States, 125 million people are living with chronic illnesses, which contribute to 70% of all deaths and one-third of years of potential life lost prior to age 65 years.

Chronic illnesses may be exacerbated by physical, psychosocial, and environmental factors that result from a disaster, including extreme temperatures, lack of food or water, physical or emotional trauma, and disruptions in the health care system. Studies evaluating the indirect mortality (that is, the mortality not directly caused by the event itself, but by the consequences of it, such as lack of access to care) of the general population after large-scale disasters have demonstrated that those with chronic medical conditions, along with women and children, are disproportionately affected. Given that approximately 80% of adults aged 65 years or older have at least one chronic medical condition and about 50% have at least two chronic conditions, this fast-growing segment of the US population is particularly vulnerable in a disaster.[6]

Circumstances faced by Hurricane Katrina survivors highlight the need for disaster planners to give priority consideration to continuity of care for persons with chronic diseases. Review of more than 21,600 patient health-related encounters in clinics one week after the hurricane found that the greatest percentage of visits was attributed to patients with chronic diseases, related conditions, and medication refills (21%), as compared to trauma (29%) and acute illness (44%).[7] In a random sample of 680 hurricane evacuees residing in a Houston shelter, researchers found that 279 (41%) had a chronic medical condition such as heart disease, hypertension, diabetes, or asthma.[8]

A survey of 1043 displaced and non-displaced Hurricane Katrina survivors (aged 18 and older) found that the majority of respondents (73.9%) had one or more chronic medical conditions during the year before the hurricane.[9] After the hurricane, more than one-fifth of respondents reported a disruption in treatment of at least one condition. Disruptions were greatest for people with mental disorders, followed by those with conditions such as diabetes and cancer. Respiratory illness, heart disease, and musculoskeletal conditions had the fewest reports of disruption. A study performed 6 months after the hurricane demonstrated a 47% increase in crude mortality in the greater New Orleans area. Researchers postulated that such a mortality increase was due to a lack of access to care for those with chronic medical conditions.[10]

A study of prescriptions filled for Hurricane Katrina survivors residing in a San Antonio evacuee center (and who received prescriptions from either the Disaster Medical Assistance Team [DMAT] pharmacy cache or from one of four retail pharmacies) disclosed the same issue of chronic disease management.[11] Thirty-eight percent of the 14,719 defined daily doses (DDD) of medications dispensed by the DMAT pharmacy were classified as chronic care medicines; 73% of the 80,424 doses provided by retail pharmacies were for chronic care. Cardiovascular medications (39%) were the most commonly dispensed DDD.

The population displaced in the aftermath of Hurricane Katrina was predominantly African American (76%), was largely unemployed or underemployed (53%), lacked health care insurance (47%), and lived with chronic health conditions (56%).[12] Approximately one-half of these evacuees lacked medications at the time of displacement. Moreover, most were not able to access their medical records in a timely fashion. Lack of access to medical records adds risks to care through incomplete medical information and inefficiency in giving care.[13] As such, evacuees have a greater risk for adverse drug events.

It is widely accepted that populations affected by natural disasters and other catastrophic emergencies experience an increase in prevalence of mental and behavioral illness between 5% and 40% (most increases are in the lower half of this range), due to the stress of human, economic, and social losses associated with such events.[14–17] The same held true for Hurricane Katrina in the New Orleans metropolitan area: there was a significant increase in the prevalence of anxiety, depression, and posttraumatic stress disorder after the storm.[17]

In sum, key lessons from Hurricane Katrina include the need for planners to identify population demographics and geography and to anticipate nonacute health care needs.

4.5 HEALTH SYSTEM PREPAREDNESS FOR DISASTERS AND PUBLIC HEALTH EMERGENCIES[18,19]

Health system preparedness involves the development of resources and organizational capacity to prevent or manage the effects of a disaster event on the basis of local risk assessments. Preparedness is a key element of disaster planning and involves all of the actions required in advance to establish and sustain the level of capability necessary to execute a wide range of disaster management operations involving the public and private sectors. Preparedness plans describe how personnel, equipment, and other governmental and nongovernmental resources will be used to support incident management requirements. Plans provide mechanisms for setting priorities, integrating multiple entities and functions, requesting disaster assistance from state and federal authorities, establishing collaborative relationships, and ensuring that communications and other systems support the full spectrum of incident management activities.

To prepare effectively, local health officials should work with other community stakeholders to integrate and coordinate community and regional disaster management plans. This involves:

➤ Conducting disaster training and education.

➤ Performing hazard vulnerability and risk assessments.

➤ Mapping specific locations of potential disasters.

➤ Taking inventory of existing health resources and assessing the ability to mobilize those resources in an emergency (ie, surge capacity planning).

➤ Designating alternate care facilities and shelters.

➤ Providing medical and mental health services, including procedures for meeting community needs when local resources are overwhelmed, damaged, or disrupted.

➤ Providing mechanisms for managing and distributing inventories of countermeasures that might be needed for various threat scenarios (eg, if mass clinics are needed, thousands of volunteers will be required, preferably coming from preexisting organized volunteer groups).

➤ Conducting both functional and field exercises to test the system for community-wide, fully integrated, disaster medical and public health response.

Health care system preparedness depends on a strong and flexible public health system at the local, state, and federal levels, and on the vigilance of health care workers, who may be the first to observe and report unusual illnesses or injuries. The capacity of the health care system to prepare and respond effectively to a serious emergency is often depicted as the pyramid of public health system preparedness (Figure 4-1)[18]:

➤ The tip of the pyramid represents public health actions taken to prevent and control injury, disease, and disability.

➤ The middle section consists of the essential public health capabilities (ie, surveillance, education and training, laboratory practice, and epidemic

FIGURE 4-1
Pyramid of Public Health
Preparedness[18]

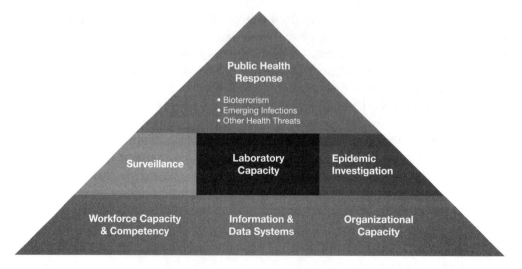

investigation) that need to be in place to support public health emergency response efforts and activities.

➤ The base of the pyramid is the basic public health infrastructure, which provides the systems, workforce, relationships, and resources to enable and sustain the performance of public health's core functions and essential services in every community.

The public health infrastructure protects the nation against the spread of disease, and from environmental and occupational hazards. It is composed of three interrelated components: a competent workforce, robust information systems, and strong organizational capacities.

4.5.1 Health Workforce Capacity and Competency

The public health system relies on a well-trained and competent workforce, including the expertise of professionals in federal, tribal, state, and local public health agencies. The broad spectrum of professionals involved in public health includes nurses, physicians, dentists, mental health specialists, epidemiologists, statisticians, health educators, environmental health specialists, industrial hygienists, food and drug inspectors, toxicologists, laboratory technicians, veterinarians, pharmacists, economists, social scientists, attorneys, nutritionists, social workers, administrators, and managers. They work not only in governmental agencies but also in clinics, health centers, academic institutions, community-based organizations, and private corporations. Working together, health professionals are trained to recognize emerging health problems and to prevent and control injuries and disease. In a bioterrorist attack, a skilled health workforce is critical to the detection of the disease outbreak, monitoring its effects, mobilizing a coordinated effort to control the spread of the disease, and studying the impact of the outbreak to inform future response efforts.

4.5.2 Health Information and Data Systems

A second component of the public health infrastructure is a robust information and communication system. Timely, credible, and reliable information is essential before, during, and after a disaster strikes. This includes up-to-date guidelines, recommendations, health alerts, and modern, standards-based information systems that monitor data on injuries and diseases and enable efficient communication among public and private health organizations, the media, and the public.

Effective information and communications systems are vital for disease surveillance. These link initially rare events to a common source, and then communicate this information quickly to frontline workers. An example is a surveillance system that assesses increased emergency department visits related to "flu-like illnesses" or other syndromes that could be related to a bioterrorism event or emerging infectious disease. By detecting an outbreak early, preventive measures can be initiated earlier, mitigating the effect of the disaster.

4.5.3 Health Organizational Capacity

A strong organizational capacity through a systems approach gives public health entities the ability to use tools, information, and personnel more effectively. This involves the consortium of public health departments and laboratories, working with private sector agencies, volunteer organizations, health care facilities, and businesses to provide essential disaster health services.

4.6 HEALTH SYSTEM RESPONSE TO DISASTERS AND PUBLIC HEALTH EMERGENCIES[20-24]

Immediate response to a disaster or other emergency involves the activation, mobilization, and deployment of community assets. When disasters exceed local, regional, and state response capacity, state governors have the authority to declare the need for federal disaster assistance via the Robert T. Stafford Disaster Relief and Emergency Assistance Act of 1988 (Public Law 93-288), available at http://www.fema.gov/about/stafact.shtm. Once this declaration is made, the Department of Homeland Security (DHS), as defined by the Homeland Security Act of 2002, assumes responsibility as the coordinating lead agency for all federal disaster response efforts. DHS defines federal disasters as incidents of national significance that meet criteria stated in the National Response Framework (NRF).

The NRF (www.fema.gov/emergency/nrf/) identifies 15 emergency support functions (ESFs), which include mechanisms for providing disaster support to states and communities. As defined by the NRF, ESF-8, Public Health and Medical Services, is coordinated by the Department of Health and Human Services (HHS), principally through the Assistant Secretary for Public Health Emergency Preparedness. The purpose of ESF-8 is to provide federal assistance to supplement state and local resources in responding to public health and medical care needs after a disaster or a public health emergency. Again, these resources are provided when state and local assets are overwhelmed *and* federal assistance has been requested. Key provisions of ESF-8 are found in the Appendix to this chapter.

4.6.1 Activation of the Local Health Emergency Response System

In a federally declared disaster, government authorities at all levels will shift from existing day-to-day organizational structures into an emergency management structure that is consistent with the National Incident Management System (NIMS). An incident commander will be appointed, as will four section chiefs to oversee efforts related to planning, operations, logistics, and finance.

Application of the incident management framework to the local medical and public health response is essential to enable appropriate communication and coordination across response agencies and to reduce morbidity and mortality. The application of NIMS for individual health care facilities is made operational through the Hospital Incident Command System. As the event becomes more widespread, it is essential for hospitals and other health care facilities to work with each other, as well as with the local public health system, to maximize the greatest good for the greatest number of casualties.

Recognizing the challenge of integrating and coordinating health-related assets in a disaster, a six-layered approach to health and medical management has been proposed.[25] As described in Chapter 3, this tiered response begins with individual hospitals. Depending on the scope and magnitude of the event, hospital assets may be augmented through community health care coalitions, local jurisdictions, state response agencies, interstate resources, and federal response agencies. When it is deemed that activities of a given tier are insufficient, then assistance from the next layer is requested. Conceptually, this tiered approach is sensible; operationalizing it within the NIMS framework can be challenging because of variations at local, county, and state jurisdictional levels.

4.6.2 Health Emergency Operations Center (HEOC)

The Health Resources and Services Administration supports the creation of health care coalitions and geographically regionalized health care systems to enhance community preparedness. Consistent with the NIMS framework, in some regions, health care organizations and institutions are working with the local public health authorities to form Health Emergency Operations Centers (HEOCs). These regional entities can be activated in disasters and public health emergencies to coordinate local health care assets in the private and public sector, and provide additional regional support for the response.[26]

Components of an HEOC include the local public health agency, local health care coalitions, relevant private sector response entities (eg, American Red Cross, Medical Reserve Corps), and state and federal partners. In addition to local medical and public health expertise, the HEOC also involves a cadre of legal and ethical experts who assist in critical decision making about resource allocation.

The main functions of the HEOC are to ensure:

➤ Situational awareness and surveillance.

➤ Population-based triage decisions and protocols.

➤ Risk communication and interventions enforcement.

➤ Resource allocation and coordination.

➤ Volunteer mobilization and just-in-time training.

➤ Monitoring health recovery systems.

FIGURE 4-2

Health Emergency
Operations Center[26]

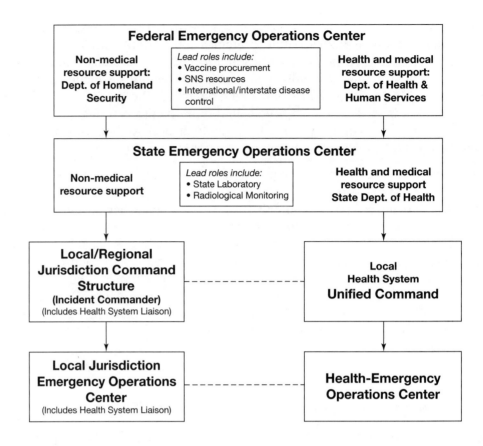

Model HEOCs have been established in Houston (Catastrophic Emergency Operations Center) and in Los Angeles. HEOCs are part of the incident command structure and promote better vertical integration of health and medical response (Figure 4-2).

Large-scale disasters and public health emergencies inherently cause a scarcity of available resources and disproportionately impact at-risk populations (eg, pregnant women, children, those with chronic disease, the elderly, the disabled, and the dispossessed). As discussed in Chapters 2 and 3, population-based triage and surge capacity management are systematic processes that recognize all potential points of contact between casualties and the available health care system.[27,28] This process is inherently dynamic, with casualty prioritization based on the accuracy and timeliness of situational awareness, the availability of resources, and the efficacy of risk communication. Population-based triage recognizes that overall mortality and morbidity are dependent on the accuracy and interoperability of four distinct stages of casualty population contact: at the community level through risk communication; at the prehospital level; at the hospital level; and at the regional/state level.

In disasters and public health emergencies, HEOCs can readily establish and maintain situational awareness to guide population-based triage and surge capacity decision making. This "macroscopic" view estimates the magnitude of the event, which includes the total numbers of deaths, injured casualties, and uninjured, at-risk people, as well as the total health care resources consumed and available. Ensuring timely and accurate situational awareness is critical for developing effective strategies, decisions, and response actions. Situational awareness is obtained through data collected via surveillance programs and survey assessments of affected communities and health care facilities. Information can be analyzed at the HEOC to guide decisions for the requisition, procurement, and deployment of resources.

HEOC personnel use "measures of effectiveness" to monitor the success or failure of the response. Such measures may include:

➤ Timeliness and accuracy of the mobilized health information system.

➤ Decline in mortality and morbidity in affected jurisdictions.

➤ Equitable surge capacity distribution for the entire population requiring care.

➤ Control of the transmissibility or reproduction rate (R0) of a communicable disease (the R0 rate refers to the average number of secondary cases of a disease generated by a typical primary case in a susceptible population; an R0 rate of 1.0 indicates no transmission).

4.6.3 Community Health System Coordination

In a serious health emergency, state and local health departments, hospitals, and other health care entities should participate as part of a coordinated and seamless response with other community emergency response sectors to protect public health and safety, restore essential services, and provide emergency relief. Depending on the incident management system that is in place for a particular situation and jurisdiction, the local public health agency can play a leading, collaborative, or supportive role. In a biologic event, to include influenza outbreaks or bioterrorism events, public and private sector health agencies will have a significant role in incident management.

Disaster response is not the responsibility of any single community agency or group. The sheer size of these events and the numbers of people involved require cooperation among numerous agencies and individuals. This includes all levels of government and private sector responders. Disaster response efforts must be "interoperable" to ensure personnel are able to work together in their appropriate response function and to avoid duplication of effort. Not only does efficiency increase; the safety of the community and responders improves as well. All potential responding and participating agencies must be aware of their roles before an event and understand how they fit into the larger disaster system.

One of the principal functions of local health care agencies, which can be achieved through the HEOC, is the coordination and distribution of medical and public health response assets to strategic locations to best meet the needs of affected communities. At the local level, these assets can be activated, mobilized, and deployed on the basis of information obtained through accurate situational assessment of populations at risk, the status of the existing regional emergency medical system capacity, the status of regional hospital and critical care bed capacity, and the local medical and public health work force. Local volunteer assets that can be utilized to assist with the immediate response include the Medical Reserve Corps and Community Emergency Response Teams.

➤ *Medical Reserve Corps (MRC)*: The MRC was created as a grassroots initiative to enhance citizen preparedness. MRC units are composed of medical and public health volunteers, such as physicians, nurses, pharmacists, dentists, veterinarians, and epidemiologists. MRCs are community-driven and exist in all states, with a volunteer base exceeding 192,000. While the MRC is not an official federal asset, its central headquarters is located within the Office of the US Surgeon General; MRC units are coordinated through that office, yet mobilization occurs locally (http://www.medicalreservecorps.gov).

➤ *Community Emergency Response Team (CERT) Program*: Administered by the Federal Emergency Management Agency (FEMA), the CERT program prepares people to help themselves, their families, and their neighbors in the event of a disaster in their community. Through CERT, citizens can learn about disaster preparedness and receive training in basic disaster response skills such as fire safety, light search and rescue, and disaster medical operations. With this training, volunteers can provide immediate assistance to casualties before first responders arrive on scene. CERT volunteers also participate in community preparedness outreach activities (http://www.citizencorps.gov/cert/index.shtm).

For large-scale disasters that exceed regional capacity, state and federal response assistance may be required. State and interstate assistance may be obtained through the Emergency Management Assistance Compact. Federal assets include the National Disaster Medical System and the Public Health Service Commissioned Corps.

➤ *Emergency Management Assistance Compact (EMAC) System*: In addition to federal response assets, a state-to-state mechanism to provide immediate medical and public health surge capacity and personnel exists through the EMAC system. The EMAC was ratified by Congress and signed into law in 1996 as an agreement among the 50 states, the District of Columbia, Puerto Rico, and the US Virgin Islands to provide state-to-state mutual aid and assistance in a disaster. EMAC offers a simplified system to expedite emergency response by allowing resources and deployed personnel from other EMAC-member states to promptly arrive at a disaster scene. After the governor of an affected area declares a state of emergency, the respective state is responsible for requesting assistance from participating EMAC states. The EMAC involves a contractual agreement for reimbursement of costs among states, as well as protection of personnel via workers' compensation and liability provisions. From medical resources to public health services to security reinforcement, EMAC allows states to share response assets efficiently for any emergency or disaster (http://www.emacweb.org/).

➤ *The National Disaster Medical System (NDMS)*: The NDMS is a federally coordinated response system that supplements state and local emergency resources during disasters or major emergencies, and provides support to the military and the Department of Veterans Affairs medical systems in caring for US casualties from overseas armed conflicts. The NDMS comprises individuals with expertise and experience in a wide range of professions, including clinical care, public health, forensics, and mortuary sciences. Response teams are positioned nationwide with personnel who have completed an application process and met prerequisite training requirements. Qualified individuals are assigned to designated teams and receive additional training in disaster management and response. NDMS personnel are required to maintain appropriate and current professional certifications and licensure in their discipline (http://www.phe.gov/ Preparedness/responders/ndms/Pages/default.aspx).

Opportunities to serve in the NDMS include:

➤ Disaster Medical Assistance Teams (including special teams for pediatrics, burns, search and rescue, and mental health).

➤ Disaster Mortuary Operational Response Teams.

➤ National Pharmacy Response Teams.

➤ National Veterinary Response Teams.

➤ *The Public Health Services Commission Corps (PHSCC):* In January 2006, the HHS secretary announced an initiative to increase PHSCC personnel by 10% to 6600 members to improve federal response operations and the deployment process, which would enable it to address public health challenges more quickly and efficiently. Such action was intended to enable the Commissioned Corps to meet its critical mission to treat disease, ensure the safety of food and medicine, and restore health and hope in times of greatest need; respond rapidly to urgent public health emergencies; fill isolated or hazardous public health positions; and meet essential federal and state level public health leadership and service roles.

In response to recommendations in the White House after-action report, *The Federal Response to Hurricane Katrina: Lessons Learned,*[2] the PHSCC developed a four-tiered public health response system:

➤ Tier 1 involves a newly created Rapid Deployment Force (RDF), which will be located and staffed strategically in multiple locations and for rapid mobilization and deployment across the nation. Tier 1 personnel will be expected to report to a point of departure within 12 hours of notification.

➤ Tier 2 involves "applied public health and mental health teams," who also will be strategically located for rapid deployment across the nation. Tier 2 personnel will be expected to depart within 36 hours of notification.

➤ Tier 3 consists of officers not placed in tiers 1 or 2; they will be expected to report within 72 hours of notification.

➤ Tier 4 consists of officers in the PHSCC inactive reserve, with no specified time requirement for their departure on notification.

In addition to this tiered response system, the PHSCC is working on a Public Health Service Health and Medical Response (HAMR) Team. Under this concept, the PHSCC would create and maintain a cadre of full-time, equipped teams dedicated to training for and responding to public health emergencies.

4.7 CRITICAL COMMUNITY HEALTH SYSTEM CAPABILITIES

In a disaster or public health emergency, health system response involves time-sensitive actions to save lives and property, as well as actions to begin stabilizing the situation to help the community cope with the situation. Community health resources will likely be challenged by a surge of people seeking treatment, prophylaxis, or decontamination. To meet this challenge, health authorities should implement various measures to control the situation and help prevent further harm. Critical public health actions include supplying of basic life-sustaining commodities, such as food, water, and shelter; enhanced surveillance; distribution of vaccines and medications; implementation of environmental controls; legal interventions to restrict the movement of affected populations; emergency risk communication; and provision of essential treatment and preventive clinical services.

4.7.1 Surveillance and Epidemiologic Investigation

Public health surveillance is the systematic, ongoing assessment of the health of a community. It provides a baseline description of a health problem and the ways in which it changes or evolves. Surveillance is a fundamental public health activity directed at all threats, whether occurring naturally or caused deliberately. The basic requirements of surveillance include trained personnel, effective reporting systems, laboratory capabilities, and communication links between various components and partners. Well-designed public health surveillance systems provide essential data to support epidemiologic investigation and inform public health decision making.

On the basis of surveillance data, investigators study unexpected or unexplained clusters of disease, detect previously unknown risk factors, develop new community prevention services, and improve intervention strategies. Well-developed surveillance and epidemiologic expertise not only facilitate initial disease detection and control but are essential to monitoring the impact of a public health emergency event, managing public concern, and evaluating the efficacy of public health responses.

Goals of Public Health Surveillance

Public health surveillance provides information to:

➤ Ensure accurate diagnosis and appropriate treatment of an individual with a disease, injury, or condition of public health importance.

➤ Identify and address the cause of the problem.

➤ Monitor the health status and trends in the community.

➤ Determine the need for and effectiveness of public health programs at the community level.

Effective surveillance is directly linked to health emergency response. Public health authorities must have the capacity to respond rapidly and act on emerging information with the full range of necessary tools. These include the legal framework for action, as well as adequate medical care facilities and treatment capabilities. Effective surveillance must be linked to emerging knowledge and technologies. This involves the need for better diagnostics to clarify the cause of the health threat quickly—including both environmental rapid detection devices and sensitive laboratory tests for human exposure and infection.

Disease surveillance systems are usually population-based and can be either active (eg, calling hospitals to locate cases) or passive (eg, mailing reports of infectious diseases to the health department). Syndromic surveillance is an emerging area of active surveillance that offers a more "real-time" alerting system than traditional disease reporting (which occurs in the context of established diagnosed disease). With this system, public health agencies and first responders may be able to deliver more aggressive, timely, and clinically relevant treatment based on syndromic categories (such as burns and trauma, respiratory failure, cardiovascular shock, and neurologic toxicity). Tracking the sale of medications (both over-the-counter and prescription) or unexplained deaths (both human and animal) are other innovative approaches to health surveillance. As demonstrated by the West Nile virus experience, monitoring for dead birds is a sentinel indicator of an emergency situation that could affect people.

During a disaster, public health surveillance activities increase dramatically and are designed to:

➤ Reduce immediate injury, illness, and death associated with the event.

➤ Document exposures.

➤ Work with physicians and other health professionals to identify people with exposure-related illnesses and injuries.

➤ Monitor long-term medical and mental health of affected individuals and populations.

➤ Determine when it is safe to return to the affected area.

Large-scale disasters and public health emergencies can cause significant damage to the public health infrastructure and surveillance systems, causing widespread population displacement and a lack of access to care. Secondary effects to both the public health system and its infrastructure contribute to the indirect mortality and morbidity of the community and can surpass direct mortality; such effects are seen particularly in complex humanitarian disasters. The devastation caused by Hurricane Katrina resulted in 1500 deaths that could be directly attributed to the storm. Six months after the event, the crude death rate in New Orleans increased 47%, accounting for 3300 deaths.[10] Subsequently, state and local health authorities have enhanced surveillance systems to monitor for further increases in physical, mental, and behavioral problems.

Surveillance systems can be established in sentinel sites (shelters, hospitals, and clinics) to monitor the health of affected populations, manage public concern, and gauge the effectiveness of ongoing relief programs. In a disease outbreak, public health officials will utilize active surveillance measures to try to locate infected and exposed persons. This includes personal calls to health care professionals in the community, and "shoe leather epidemiology," through which public health employees contact infected people and interview family members to identify contacts and other ill or exposed people. Results of ongoing surveillance and assessment activities are used to modify relief efforts as appropriate.

An essential aspect of any public health surveillance program is assurance that the privacy rights of people whose information is of interest will not be violated. All states have statutes or regulations that provide some level of privacy protection for individual medical records and for health-related data maintained by the government. The conflict between the right to privacy and the need to know concerning health data must be monitored and addressed by any health surveillance program and is covered in existing federal legislation. For public health surveillance, the Health Insurance Portability and Accountability Act of 1996 (HIPAA) allows for the disclosure of patient data to appropriate authorities.[29,30]

4.7.2 Rapid Needs Assessment

A key initial step in mobilizing a disaster response for an affected population is to obtain information about the extent of the population's immediate needs and the status of the supporting health infrastructure. A rapid needs assessment (RNA) is performed to obtain objective and reliable information that describes a population's specific needs for emergency relief services. This includes the extent of the required response and areas where specialized assistance is needed.

RNA teams are usually deployed to the disaster area 3 to 10 days after the event. These teams interview people in their homes about their needs. Households to be interviewed (approximately 200) are selected by statistical sampling to accurately assess community needs, and information is collected on a one-page standardized survey. Geographic information systems can assist with population-based sampling and are being used in the response to large-scale natural disasters and complex humanitarian emergencies. RNAs monitor mortality rates, usually as crude rates, by querying local civic leaders or local health facilities. RNA teams also can assess availability of and access to essential services such as water, food, shelter, electric power, transportation, medications, and other supplies. The collected data can be used to guide disaster response efforts to meet the identified needs of the community.

4.7.3 Emergency Risk Communication

Getting accurate information to people quickly is a key component to saving lives during a disaster. Crisis and emergency risk communication provides information for individuals, stakeholders, or an entire community as a way to support the best possible decisions to protect their health. During emergencies, the public may receive information from a variety of sources. Effective communication of clear, concise, and credible information may reassure the public that the situation is being addressed competently. Effective public information must reach broad audiences to publicize both immediate and anticipated health hazards, appropriate health and safety precautions, the need for evacuation, and alternative travel routes. The media can play an important role in this regard by keeping the public informed, as these examples illustrate:

➤ A hurricane or flood contaminates the city water supply, and residents need to avoid direct consumption until appropriate decontamination is performed.

➤ Smoke from a large forest fire or ash from a volcano increases atmospheric particulate contamination in the area, posing a risk to people with respiratory conditions.

➤ A severe influenza outbreak places thousands of citizens at risk, particularly the very old and the very young. Immunization stations may need to be established, and the media, through the use of appropriate physician consultation, may provide advice on appropriate precautions, the location of available immunization stations, and contact information for those who require prophylaxis or care.

Under NIMS, state and local health authorities must have established procedures for providing the news media with timely and accurate public information. One way to ensure coordination of public information is by establishing a Joint Information Center (JIC). Using the JIC as a central location, information can be coordinated and integrated across jurisdictions and agencies, and among all government partners, the private sector, and nongovernmental agencies. In many respects, the JIC is the information analog to health with the HEOC.

In a disaster, public health officials will need to give citizens necessary and appropriate information and involve them in making decisions that affect their health, safety, and well-being. Sound and thoughtful risk communication can assist public officials in preventing ineffective, fear-driven, and potentially damaging public responses to serious events like unusual disease outbreaks and acts of terrorism. Moreover, appropriate risk communication can foster public trust and confidence. During a disaster, the aims of risk communication are to[31]:

➤ Help people more accurately understand their own risks.

➤ Provide background information and reassurance to affected individuals and populations by answering these questions:

   ➤ How could this happen?

   ➤ Has this happened before?

   ➤ How can I prevent this from happening again?

   ➤ Will I be all right in the long term—will I recover?

➤ Gain understanding and support for response and recovery plans.

➤ Listen to stakeholder and audience feedback and correct misinformation.

➤ Explain emergency recommendations.

➤ Empower risk/benefit decision making.

The redundant delivery of information through several sources can help to fill communication gaps in the event of power outages or other interruptions in services. Specific risk communication venues include:

➤ Toll-free information telephone lines (such as community hotlines).

➤ Electronic information services.

➤ Radio, television, newspaper, and Internet news sites.

➤ Briefings and press conferences.

➤ Community mailings (flyers and newsletters).

➤ Public meetings.

While the media can reach large numbers of people, there are many groups in the United States that do not have ready access to mass communication channels in an emergency. Potential barriers that can severely hamper the ability to receive and act on relevant health/risk information in a disaster include:

➤ Lack of access to television, radio, Internet, telephone, or other typical communication venues.

➤ Cognitive impairments.

➤ Language/linguistic barriers.

➤ Physical impairments (blindness, deafness).

➤ Preexisting psychological conditions.

➤ Preexisting political/legal conditions (undocumented residency status, child support defaults, mistrust of the organization sending the information).

➤ Homelessness.

➤ Strongly held cultural and religious beliefs and customs that run counter to recommended actions (eg, mandatory vaccination).

CDC Crisis and Emergency Risk Communication Resources

The Centers for Disease Control and Prevention (CDC) uses a variety of information resources to communicate accurate information about public health threats:

➤ *Public Information Contact Center and Clinician Information Line (CDC-INFO or 800-232-4636):* The CDC maintains a toll-free public information contact center to ensure that the general public, clinicians, and emergency responders have a number to call and obtain information during a public health emergency.

➤ *Clinician Outreach and Communication Activity (http://www.bt.cdc.gov/coca/).* To facilitate the rapid dissemination of information to clinicians, the CDC operates the Clinician Outreach and Communication Activity (COCA). The CDC sends weekly e-mail updates on emergency preparedness and response topics to the 40,000 individual members and 145 partner health and medical organizations. The CDC also announces new training opportunities related to emergency preparedness and response topics to clinician members.

➤ *Emergency Preparedness and Response website (http://www.emergency.cdc.gov).* This website provides updated content on natural disasters, terrorist events, national emergencies, and outbreaks within a half-hour of newly released information. Targeted information can be accessed by critical audiences such as the general public, first responders, clinicians, scientists, and the state and local public health workforce. The website contains resources on more than 100 emergency topics.

➤ *Health Alert Network (http://www2a.cdc.gov/han/Index.asp):* The Health Alert Network (HAN) is a nationwide program that links local health departments and other organizations to disseminate critical information on urgent health threats and appropriate response. The HAN helps ensure that communities have rapid and timely access to emergent health information and evidence-based practices for effective public health preparedness and response on a 24 hours/day, 7 days/week basis.

➤ *Translation Services for Emergency Information:* The CDC can translate information and emergency requests into more than 75 languages. This translation capability enables the CDC to provide appropriate communications to a variety of populations in a disaster. Other available services include interpretation, signing, and voice-over in Spanish for any audio or video files.

The CDC Crisis and Emergency Risk Communication website includes resources and online courses designed for personnel who perform crisis and risk communication, as well as media relations, in a disaster or public health emergency. Target audiences include federal, state, and local public health professionals; health care professionals; emergency medical services professionals; and civic and community leaders. For more information, see http://www.bt.cdc.gov/cerc.

4.7.4 Communicable Disease Control

Disaster conditions can facilitate disease transmission and increase susceptibility to infection. Disease outbreaks can result from breakdowns in environmental safeguards, crowding in temporary shelters or camps, malnutrition, inadequate surveillance, and limited availability of medical treatment services. Communicable diseases can be transmitted directly person-to-person or indirectly through contaminated food and water, or disease vectors (insects or rodents). Disease pathogens that can be transmitted through contact with human feces include *Escherichia coli*, *Salmonella* sp, *Shigella* sp, and hepatitis viruses, as well as third-world conditions such as typhoid fever, cholera, bacillary and amoebic dysentery, schistosomiasis, and various helminthic infestations.

Public health officials should monitor the situation closely and implement measures to prevent or limit the spread of infectious diseases. Such measures include:

➤ Sanitation (adequate waste disposal, food protection, provision of clean water, and vector control).

➤ Medical intervention (vaccination, laboratory services, case management, adequate nutrition).

➤ Public health surveillance.

4.7.5   Environmental Health Services

In a disaster, health authorities provide for the monitoring and evaluation of environmental health risks or hazards and ensure that appropriate actions are taken to protect the health and safety of responders and affected populations. With biologic events, prevention of disease spread, rather than identification and management of individual casualties, is the primary goal. Postdisaster environmental health efforts include:

➤ Environmental monitoring and surveillance.

➤ Inspection of the purity and usability of foodstuffs, water, drugs, and other consumables that were exposed to the hazard.

➤ Basic sanitation.

➤ Adequate shelter.

➤ Vector control (control of insects and rodents).

➤ Remediation of contaminated environments.

Health department officials should coordinate with water, public works, and sanitation departments to ensure the availability of potable water, an effective sewage system, and sanitary garbage disposal, as well as to prevent the discharge of contaminated water, soil, and waste into water sources used for consumption or agriculture.

Potable water may be needed for drinking, cooking, and personal hygiene. Health authorities at disaster sites must plan for additional water to support clinical facilities, feeding centers, and other public health activities. Relief efforts to reduce morbidity and mortality also involve communicable disease control and restoration of proper nutritional resources. In addition to food and water (see Sphere Project box below), shelter is often the most immediate need of disaster-stricken populations.

The Sphere Project

In 1997, an international initiative, called the Sphere Project, was created to develop minimum standards for mass care in core areas of humanitarian assistance. These minimum standards seek to quantify requirements for such basic needs as water, sanitation, food and nutrition, shelter, and health care. The standards provide a framework for public health priorities and intervention in any disaster or public health emergency. The Sphere Project (http://www.sphereproject.org) is based on two core beliefs: first, that all possible steps should be taken to alleviate human suffering arising out of calamity and conflict, and second, that those affected by disaster have a right to life with dignity and therefore a right to assistance.

Selected minimum humanitarian standards are as follows:

➤ Food: 2100 kcal/day.

➤ Water: 2.5 to 3 L/day for drinking; 15 L/day for daily cleaning.

➤ Toilets (in feeding centers): one toilet per 50 adults; one toilet per 20 children.

➤ Shelter space: minimum surface area of 45 m^2 for each person; the initial covered floor area per person is at least 3.5 m^2.

Proper management of human waste is a public health priority during a disaster. Sanitation efforts are focused on reducing fecal contamination of food and water supplies to control the spread of infectious disease. Adequate sanitary facilities must be provided for affected individuals and emergency response personnel. If required, actions must be taken to prevent or control vectors such as flies, mosquitoes, and rodents, and to inspect damaged buildings for health hazards.

4.7.6   Laboratory Testing and Analysis

Various hospital, commercial, and public health laboratories support public health surveillance activities.[32] These entities provide for the definitive identification of biologic and chemical agents; such identification assists medical and public health authorities with the design and implementation of appropriate disease prevention and control measures.

Agency for Toxic Substances and Disease Registry (ATSDR)

Located within the CDC, the ATSDR performs specific functions concerning the effect of hazardous substances in the environment on public health. These functions include public health assessments of waste sites, health consultations concerning specific hazardous substances, health surveillance and registries, response to emergency releases of hazardous substances, applied research in support of public health assessments, information development and dissemination, and education and training concerning hazardous substances. For more information, see http://www.atsdr.cdc.gov.

To enhance diagnostic capacity, the CDC, health departments, and the Association of Public Health Laboratories established the Laboratory Response Network (LRN), composed of local, state, and federal laboratories. The LRN facilitates sample collection, transport, testing, and training for laboratory readiness.[33] All 50 state public health laboratories are registered members of the LRN (or are covered by a neighboring state public health laboratory). The LRN plays an important role as well in educating and training laboratory workers about safety precautions and appropriate test procedures for potential biologic and chemical terrorism agents and other rare or emerging infectious disease agents.

Laboratory testing is needed to determine whether a "flu-like illness" may be due to influenza, anthrax, or some other cause, and whether the disease agent is susceptible to available medications. State and local health authorities have a responsibility to ensure access to laboratory services for diagnostic testing that supports emergency health and medical services in a time-sensitive manner. Many local agencies and medical facilities, however, lack the resources and expertise to perform specialized diagnostic tests (eg, bioterrorism agents). The LRN fills this void.

LRN Structure for Biologic Testing: LRN labs are designated as either national, reference, or sentinel. Designation depends on the types of tests a laboratory can perform and how it handles infectious agents to protect workers and the public. About 150 state, territorial, and community public health laboratories are members of the biologic component of the LRN network:

➤ *National laboratories* have unique resources to handle highly infectious agents and the ability to identify specific agent strains. National laboratories, including those operated by the CDC, US Army Medical Research Institute for Infectious Diseases, and the Naval Medical Research Center, are responsible for specialized strain characterizations, bioforensics, and handling of highly infectious biologic agents.

➤ *Reference laboratories* can perform tests to detect and confirm the presence of many disease pathogens. These laboratories are designed and equipped to ensure a timely local response in the event of a bioterrorist incident. Rather than having to rely on confirmation from the CDC, reference laboratories are capable of producing definitive results, which then allows local authorities to respond more quickly to potential outbreaks and emergencies. There are more than 100 reference laboratories in the United States across local public health, military, veterinary, agriculture, food, and water testing facilities.

➤ *Sentinel laboratories* represent the thousands of hospital-based laboratories that are on the front lines of disease surveillance. They have a key role in the early detection of biologic agents but may not be equipped to perform more specialized testing as reference laboratories. In an unannounced or covert bioterrorist attack, patients would provide specimens during routine clinical care. Sentinel laboratories that detect a suspicious pathogen would refer the isolate to the appropriate reference laboratory.

The LRN is working with state public health laboratory directors to ensure that the estimated 25,000 private and commercial laboratories in the United States are part of the LRN. Most of these laboratories are located in hospitals, clinics, and commercial diagnostic facilities.

LRN Structure for Chemical Testing: Currently, 62 state, territorial, and metropolitan public health laboratories are members of the chemical component of the LRN network. A designation of Level 1, 2, or 3 defines network participation, and each level builds on the preceding level.

➤ *Level 3 laboratories* comprise all chemical LRN network members. These facilities are responsible for:

  ➢ Working with hospitals in their jurisdiction.

  ➢ Knowing how to properly collect and ship clinical specimens.

  ➢ Ensuring that specimens, which can be used as evidence in a criminal investigation, are handled properly and that chain-of-custody procedures are followed.

  ➢ Being familiar with chemical agents and their health effects.

  ➢ Training on anticipated clinical sample flow and shipping regulations.

  ➢ Working to develop a coordinated response plan for their respective state and jurisdiction.

➤ *Level 2 laboratories* have personnel trained to detect exposure to a limited number of toxic chemical agents in human blood or urine. Analysis of cyanide and various metals in human samples are examples of Level 2 laboratory capabilities.

➤ *Level 1 laboratories* have personnel trained to detect exposure to an expanded number of chemicals in human blood or urine, including all Level 2 laboratory analyses, plus analyses for mustard agents, nerve agents, and other highly toxic chemicals.

Biosafety Level Classifications

All US laboratories that work with biologic agents are rated according to a biosafety level (BSL) classification system. Levels range from 1 to 4, with level 1 being the lowest level of proficiency. BSL classification is used to determine the types of agents scientists can work with, the extent of testing they can perform, and the safety precautions that must be in place to protect workers and prevent the release of potentially dangerous microorganisms into the environment.

➤ *BSL-1* laboratories are used to study agents not known to consistently cause disease in healthy adult humans, and that pose minimal potential hazard to laboratory personnel and the environment. Researchers are required to follow basic safety procedures and require no special equipment or design features.

(continued)

➤ *BSL-2* laboratories are used to study agents that pose a danger if accidentally inhaled, swallowed, or exposed to the skin (eg, plague). Diseases related to these agents can be treated through available antibiotics or prevented through immunization. Safety measures include the use of protective gear such as gloves, eyewear, and lab coats, as well as handwashing sinks, waste decontamination, and safety equipment.

➤ *BSL-3* laboratories are used to study agents that can be transmitted through the air and cause potentially lethal infection (eg, West Nile virus). Researchers perform testing in air-tight enclosures. Other safety features include personal protective equipment, clothing decontamination, sealed windows, and specialized ventilation systems.

➤ *BSL-4* laboratories are used to study agents that pose a high risk of life-threatening disease for which no vaccine or therapy is available (eg, Ebola virus). Laboratory personnel must wear full-body, air-supplied suits and shower when exiting the facility. These laboratories incorporate all BSL-2 and BSL-3 features. In addition, BSL-4 laboratories are required to be negative-pressure rooms that are completely sealed and isolated to prevent release of viable agents into the environment.

More information about state public health laboratories can be accessed through the Association of Public Health Laboratories at http://www.aphl.org. Information on specimen collection and laboratory testing requirements is available on the CDC website at http://www.bt.cdc.gov/labissues/index.asp.

4.7.7   Medical Prophylaxis and Treatment

Public health authorities are responsible for developing community protocols for the care of ill and exposed casualties, as well as the disposition of remains. These include:

➤ Providing disease-specific information to the health care community on identifying cases.

➤ Issuing guidance for the clinical management of ill and exposed persons.

➤ Distributing medications to the population, including determining the locations of mass prophylaxis/treatment clinics and the logistics for staffing such clinics.

➤ Establishing Mortuary care.

For infectious diseases in which a vaccine has been developed and has been shown to be safe and effective, immunization is a key public health intervention.

Immunizations are cost-effective measures for the control of many infectious diseases, including measles, polio, tetanus, influenza, chickenpox, and pertussis. Immunizations are a vital component of the public health response for several infectious disease–related public health emergencies, including smallpox and influenza. After an initial case of smallpox, for example, public health teams should implement mass vaccination programs for the general population. The goal is to immunize the entire community within 4 days.

In addition to vaccines, public health officials will consider the use of medications to prevent or control the spread of disease. Antibiotics can be effective against the bacteria that cause plague, anthrax, and tularemia, among others. While the anthrax vaccine may have a role in postexposure prophylaxis after an anthrax event, the primary preventive measure will be antibiotic prophylaxis. For viral diseases such as influenza, various antiviral medications will be considered.

Providing medications to prevent a disease is not a new approach for public health; this is a common strategy to prevent bacterial meningitis and tuberculosis in a community. However, the urgency and scale of providing medications is significantly increased after a serious disease outbreak or act of bioterrorism. To be effective, most medications must be given to exposed people within a very short time frame. As discussed in Chapter 3, the Strategic National Stockpile (SNS) supports local and state public health agencies in the receipt and distribution of medical countermeasures and equipment.

While immediate attention will be directed to the care of sick or injured casualties, public health workers also coordinate with mortuary services to address the disposition of human remains and with animal care and control agencies for the disposal of dead animals.

4.7.8 Mental Health Services

In addition to the substantial impact that traumatic events can have on physical health, such events can create significant stress and other psychological problems for affected individuals, families, disaster responders, and relief workers. Public health response efforts should include provisions for identifying and obtaining services for affected people to reduce the occurrence and severity of adverse mental health outcomes.

Health care response efforts should include provisions for identifying and obtaining mental health services for those affected by an emergency situation. Public health authorities have a role in:

➤ Helping restore the psychological and social functioning of individuals and the community.

➤ Reducing the occurrence and severity of adverse mental health outcomes in affected populations.

➤ Ensuring that appropriate mental health resources are available for affected populations, emergency responders, and disaster managers during response and recovery operations. This includes crisis counseling, screening, diagnostic, and treatment services.

➤ Assisting with public information and risk communication efforts.

➤ Developing public information and education strategies and materials on mental health consequences of disasters. This includes providing information about normal reactions to disaster-related stress and how to handle those reactions.

4.7.9   Protection of At-Risk Populations

While the public health system seeks to prevent and control injury and disease in all populations, particular attention is directed to those with special health needs. The terms *at-risk*, *special needs*, and *vulnerable populations* are often used interchangeably. These terms are multidimensional and include widely diverse population groups with very different needs and capabilities to access available resources. Such populations may be difficult to identify or locate, and may be more susceptible or exposed to particular risks during or after a disaster or public health emergency. Examples include undocumented immigrants; transient populations; minorities; medically or chemically dependent people, homeless or shelter-dependent people; children, women, and the elderly; people with chronic health problems; people with limited or no English proficiency; physically or mentally disabled individuals (blind, deaf, hard of hearing, cognitive disorders, mobility limitations); and people who are geographically or culturally isolated.

In recent years, researchers have attempted to categorize the most common predictors of population vulnerability. These predictors can help to ascertain the physical and psychological impacts of disasters on specific population subgroups and enable community preparedness. Determinants of vulnerability such as gender, age, race, and ethnicity may not always be enough to identify all vulnerable populations within a specific region.

Vulnerability has many different connotations, and identifying conditions that make people vulnerable may not be always simple. In some cases, the vulnerability of population subgroups is determined by social geography or by the type of event taking place. For instance, coastal populations are considered vulnerable to environmental conditions, such as hurricanes and sea level rise. However, these subgroups may not be equally at risk if another type of event takes place. In addition, socially created vulnerabilities can change as conditions evolve.

Disaster Technical Assistance Center

Established by the Substance Abuse and Mental Health Services Administration (SAMHSA), the Disaster Technical Assistance Center (DTAC) supports SAMHSA efforts to prepare states, territories, and localities for delivery of an effective behavioral health response during disasters. The website contains a library of print and electronic resource materials to help meet disaster behavioral health needs. The Center maintains a toll-free help line (800-308-3515), a comprehensive website (http://www.mentalhealth.samhsa.gov/dtac/default .asp), and an e-mail address (dtac@esi-dc.com).

In the NDLS Program, the terms *at-risk*, *special needs*, and *vulnerable populations* are used interchangeably to characterize groups whose needs are not fully addressed by traditional service providers. Examples include:

➤ A disabled person whose needs cannot be met in a shelter.

➤ A non–English-speaking person who does not understand a mandatory evacuation order.

➤ An elderly person who lives alone and has limited mobility.

➤ A recent immigrant who is reluctant to ask for help.

4.7.10 Protection of Pediatric Populations[34–36]

The "pediatric population" constitutes several special populations—premature infants (born earlier than 36 weeks' gestation), neonates (birth to 1 month of age), infants (1 through 12 months of age), toddlers (1–2 years of age), preschoolers (3–5 years of age), school-agers (6–12 years of age), and adolescents (13–18 years of age). Each of these subgroups has distinguishing anatomic, physiologic, developmental, and behavioral characteristics that must be addressed by emergency preparedness and disaster management.

In disasters, the truism that "children are not small adults" remains valid. By weight, children breathe, drink, and eat more than adults, thereby requiring more active respiratory support, volume resuscitation, and energy intake. Oxygen, fluid, and medication dosing necessarily must correlate with body mass. The ranges of normal for pediatric vital signs, and the rapidity and time course of physiologic deterioration, are different from those of adults. Children are shorter and closer to the ground, where dense toxic gases and contaminated dust tend to accumulate; they are smaller, so they lose heat more quickly, impeding the effectiveness of resuscitative measures; and they are susceptible to bioactive vectors that would not ordinarily cause derangement in adults. All of these factors can lead to presentations of illness and injury that vary from those of adults.

One pediatric trauma patient can be challenging in hospitals that do not provide regular pediatric trauma care. Several other factors make emergency care of children more difficult during disasters:

➤ Children cannot self-identify.

➤ Children cannot provide reliable exposure histories.

➤ Children cannot effectively communicate their symptoms.

➤ Children may be afraid of strangers wearing personal protective equipment.

➤ Children may be unable to walk through decontamination lines without parental assistance.

➤ Children cannot legally consent to their medical care.

➤ Children can be an afterthought in disaster planning.

4.7.11   Providing Continuity of Care

In the wake of Hurricane Katrina, the provision of continued care for people with chronic conditions (eg, diabetes, human immunodeficiency virus [HIV]/ acquired immunodeficiency syndrome [AIDS], cardiovascular disease, cancer) became a priority health issue. Surveys of individuals and institutions involved in the delivery of health care to affected populations indicated that the most frequently mentioned barrier to providing care was maintaining continuity of medications.[37] Contributing factors included inadequate information (lack of medical records, low literacy) and financial constraints.

One effort to provide continuity of care in Hurricane Katrina involved a private-public consortium composed of the American Medical Association (AMA), Gold Standard, the Markle Foundation, RxHub, SureScripts, Louisiana Department of Health, Mississippi Department of Health, and the HHS Office of the National Coordinator for Health Information Technology. These groups came together and developed KatrinaHealth.org, an online service to provide physicians and pharmacists who were treating Hurricane Katrina evacuees with access to the evacuee prescription drug and dosage information. This allowed health care professionals to renew medications, safely prescribe additional medications, and avoid potential medication errors. KatrinaHealth. org provided authorized users with free access to the medication history and prescriptions for evacuees who lived in the areas affected by Hurricane Katrina.

The prescription information was made available from a variety of government and commercial sources, some of which have been aggregated. Sources include electronic databases from commercial pharmacies, government health insurance programs such as Medicaid, private insurers, and pharmacy benefits managers in the states affected by the storm. The AMA assisted in this initiative by providing independent confirmation of the identity of each physician seeking access to KatrinaHealth.org and by confirming that such physicians held an unrestricted current license to practice medicine in at least one state.

Because of the demand and success of KatrinaHealth.org and the concern that large-scale disasters are increasing in both magnitude and frequency, collaborating organizations in KatrinaHealth.org contributed to the creation of a new system, renamed "In Case of Emergency Prescription History Service." This service, ICERx, was discontinued on April 15, 2011. In a federally declared disaster, authorized clinicians and pharmacists could use this public service, at no cost, to view evacuee prescription histories online, obtain available patient allergy information and other alerts, view drug interaction reports, see therapeutic duplication reports, and query clinical pharmacology drug information, as long as displaced persons can recall their name and last known address. The system was accessible only to authorized health care professionals and pharmacists who were providing treatment or supporting the provision of treatment to evacuees. It was designed to assist health care providers in obtaining:

➤ Evacuee outpatient prescription history (drug name and dosage, quantity and day supply, name of pharmacy that filled the prescription, name of person who wrote the prescription).

➤ Available patient clinical alerts (drug interaction alerts, therapeutic duplication alerts, elderly alerts).

➤ Clinical Pharmacology® drug reference information (drug monographs, interaction reports, drug identifier tools).

4.8 EMERGENCY PUBLIC HEALTH POWERS

The power to implement measures necessary to protect public health in an emergency is reserved for each state under the US Constitution. These measures seek to balance individual rights and freedoms with the common welfare of the general population. In a disaster or public health emergency, states have authority to exert reasonable control over citizens to directly secure and promote the welfare of the state and its people. The power to act in the best interests of the people provides states and municipalities with broad discretion in how they respond to a disaster situation. This includes possible encroachment on civil rights of people in the affected area to promote the public welfare.

Once a disaster or an emergency situation has been declared by government authorities, there are multiple orders that may be issued on the basis of the public health powers available to the locality. These may include:

➤ Enforcing safety and sanitary codes.

➤ Conducting inspections.

➤ Requiring health care professionals to report certain diseases to state authorities.

➤ Establishing curfews.

➤ Controlling entry into and out of the community.

➤ Closing schools and businesses.

➤ Ordering the evacuation of buildings, streets, neighborhoods, and cities.

➤ Closing access to buildings, streets, or other public or private areas.

➤ Imposing travel restrictions.

➤ Controlling ingress and egress to and from a disaster area.

➤ Controlling movement of persons within a disaster area.

➤ Suspending the sale or dispensing of alcoholic beverages.

➤ Suspending or limiting the sale, dispensing, or transportation of firearms, explosives, or combustibles.

➤ Authorizing the acquisition or destruction of property, supplies, and materials.

➤ Issuing orders for the disposal of corpses.

The declaration of a public health emergency also may enable special powers to protect public health and safety. These include the power to:

➤ Implement medical protocols and procedures to limit the spread of a disease (eg, mandatory vaccinations).

➤ Isolate and quarantine persons.

➤ Access and disclose protected health information.

➤ License and appoint health care professionals.

While these measures may benefit the population in a public health emergency, state and local health authorities should review statutes, regulations, and ordinances that authorize these emergency measures and ensure legally sound procedures for executing them. It is important that the entire health community understand the legal and ethical implications of these emergency powers in order to implement them effectively and in a manner that places the least possible infringement on individual rights and liberties. These issues are discussed further in Chapter 5.

Isolation and Quarantine

Isolation and quarantine are two of the oldest public health interventions, dating back centuries. The purpose of both interventions is to decrease the number of individuals exposed to a contagious disease.

➤ *Isolation* is the placement of people known to have a communicable disease in a separate area where they will not expose others.

➤ *Quarantine* is the placement of people exposed to a contagious disease, but currently asymptomatic, in a separate area where they will not expose others and can be monitored for the development of the disease. Quarantine is required for several infectious diseases, such as tuberculosis, smallpox, and severe acute respiratory syndrome (SARS), because individuals can be contagious before the development of the signs and symptoms of the disease. During this asymptomatic but contagious period, they can potentially infect a large number of people.

4.9 MASS CARE

Under ESF-6, Mass Care, Emergency Assistance, Housing, and Human Services, the Federal Emergency Management Agency (FEMA) is designated as the primary federal agency responsible for coordinating and leading the federal response for mass care and related human services, in close coordination with states and volunteer organizations. The American Red Cross is the primary agency charged to assist FEMA with this effort. *Mass care* involves the coordination of nonmedical services to include sheltering of displaced persons, organizing feeding operations, providing emergency first aid at designated sites, collecting and providing information on casualties to family members, and coordinating bulk distribution of emergency relief items. Housing involves the provision of assistance for short- and long-term housing needs of displaced persons. Human services include counseling, identifying support for people with special needs, processing of claims, and expediting mail services in affected areas.[38] ESF-6 does not include recovery activities. As a private, nonprofit organization, the American Red Cross independently provides recovery assistance under its Congressional charter.

Founded in 1891, the American Red Cross provides domestic disaster relief and offers compassionate services in the following five areas:

➤ Community services to help the needy.

➤ Support and comfort for military members and their families.

➤ Collection, processing, and distribution of lifesaving blood and blood products.

➤ Educational programs that promote health and safety.

➤ International relief and development programs.

Red Cross services include mass sheltering, feeding, emergency first aid, bulk distribution of emergency relief items, and the collection and provision of information on disaster casualties to family members. The American Red Cross has 700 locally supported chapters that assist in providing these services.

4.10 IDENTIFICATION AND TRACKING OF CASUALTIES AND DISPLACED PERSONS

Tracking and identification of casualties and displaced people in a disaster is a challenging issue, particularly when people evacuate an affected region. After a disaster, displaced individuals may lose their medications, deplete their medication supplies, or forget what prescription drugs or dosage they are taking. Evacuees may not be able to contact their regular physician, clinic, or hospital. In some cases, paper-based medical records may have been destroyed.

Currently, no true standard casualty evacuation template exists for use at the disaster scene; therefore, most authorities use standardized triage tags as a tool for tracking. A true tracking system requires significant investment in interoperable health information systems at the federal, state, and local level, and must take into account all potential points of transfer (prehospital, facility, interfacility, nursing home, shelter). To date, these systems have occurred most effectively at county and community levels.

4.11 HEALTH SYSTEM MANAGEMENT OF PANDEMICS AND OTHER LARGE-SCALE INFECTIOUS DISEASE OUTBREAKS[39–41]

In 2009, global attention was fixed on the emergence and spread of a novel H1N1 influenza A virus. As a consequence of confirmed cases of H1N1 disease in the United States, the acting secretary of the US Department of Health and Human Services declared the existence of a public health emergency on April 26, 2009, recognizing that the H1N1 virus had significant potential to affect national security. On April 29, 2009, the World Health Organization (WHO) raised the pandemic alert level to Phase 5, signaling that a pandemic was imminent and that expedient efforts were needed to finalize the organization, communication, and implementation of planned mitigation measures. The WHO declared the flu outbreak a "public health emergency of international concern" under the International Health Regulations. On June 11, 2009, the WHO declared the existence of a global pandemic. By August 2010, when the WHO declared that the world had entered the postpandemic period, more than 200 countries and overseas territories had reported confirmed cases of pandemic H1N1 influenza with over 18,000 deaths.

Recent attention also has been focused on the spread of avian or "bird" flu across eastern Asia and other countries. This disease, caused by an H5N1 influenza virus, can infect humans and has resulted in more than 100 deaths in several countries. To date, those who have been infected were poultry workers or others who had contact with sick birds or surfaces contaminated by such birds. Health experts are concerned that the virus could change to a form that is spread easily from person to person.

Past influenza pandemics have occurred at intervals of 10 to 60 years, with three in the 20th century (1918, 1957–1958, and 1967–1968). A pandemic is a disease that has spread around the world, creating a serious public health emergency. A pandemic can occur when three conditions are met:

➤ A new disease emerges to which a population has little or no immunity.

➤ The disease is infectious for humans.

➤ The disease spreads easily among humans.

Pandemic flu is usually more serious than a typical seasonal flu. For an influenza pandemic to occur, the flu virus must undergo a major change that essentially results in a new form of the virus that, while more virulent, is also more transmissible. This "new" virus is not recognized by the immune systems of most people, leaving them with little natural resistance. The large pool of susceptible people allows the virus to spread broadly and rapidly, thus creating the potential for a serious public health emergency. Further, pandemic flu differs from seasonal flu in that it has the potential to infect populations of *different ages* globally.

In a pandemic, large numbers of infected people and those who believe they may be infected will overwhelm community health systems. There may simply not be enough resources to take care of everyone who thinks they need emergency care. Resources such as ventilators and medications may need to be allocated according to publicly accepted protocols. In such situations, difficult decisions will need to be made regarding who gets these resources, including vaccines.

An important secondary impact of a serious pandemic is societal disruption. Impacts can range from school and business closings to the interruption of basic services in public transportation and food delivery. Institutions, such as schools and workplaces, may close because a large proportion of students or employees are ill. Essential services may be limited because workers are absent. Travel between cities and countries may be sharply reduced, not only due to fewer workers available to operate transportation systems, but because fewer people travel. An especially severe pandemic could lead to serious illness and increased death rates (even among young and healthy people), social disorder, and economic loss. Large numbers of people in many places would become seriously ill simultaneously.

In 1918, an influenza pandemic killed 675,000 people in the United States and 20 to 50 million people around the world. In 2003, an outbreak of SARS caused economic losses and social disruption far beyond the affected countries and well out of proportion to the number of cases and deaths. While influenza is distinctly different from SARS, a pandemic of similar severity would have a similarly disruptive effect on societies and economies.

4.11.1 Preparation and Planning

Prevention is the foundation for the entire spectrum of pandemic preparedness activities, including surveillance, detection, containment, and response. Prevention requires pre-pandemic commitment to:

➤ Develop and exercise pandemic preparedness and response plans.

➤ Invest in pharmaceutical research and development to ensure capacity to produce, deliver, and stockpile vaccines and medications.

➤ Expand domestic and global public health, clinical, veterinary, and scientific capacity to track illness patterns and respond to an outbreak.

➤ Educate populations about high-risk practices that increase the likelihood of disease transmission.

> ➤ Develop mechanisms to recruit and deploy rapidly large numbers of public health, clinical, veterinary, and other health professionals within or across jurisdictions to meet health-related needs.

> ➤ Communicate expectations and responsibilities with stakeholders and the public.

A critical element of pandemic planning is to help people and organizations not accustomed to responding to a health crisis to understand the actions and priorities required to prepare for and respond to a large-scale disease outbreak. Those groups include political leadership at all levels of government, non-health government agencies, and non-health members of the private sector. Essential planning also includes coordination of efforts between human and veterinary health authorities.

Pandemic preparedness activities largely involve assessing capacities and capabilities for dealing with the expected surge in demand for supplies and resources. In combination with traditional public health measures, vaccines and medications are the foundation of a national infection control strategy. Attention must be given to establishing medication and vaccine production capacity and stockpiles in support of national containment and response strategies. Pandemic planning requires that health authorities assess possible control measures; drug and vaccine inventories; emergency mechanisms to increase drug and vaccine supplies; legal and liability issues for mass prophylaxis; and research, development, and production capacities for new drugs and vaccines.

State and local preparedness plans should contain clear guidelines on setting priorities for the use of scarce resources such as vaccines, drugs, ventilators, and hospital beds. To avoid overwhelming hospitals, community pandemic plans need to provide for the establishment of alternate care facilities (such as schools) to treat sick and exposed people. Community plans should also address the great need for local volunteers to work in these facilities because most health care personnel will remain in hospitals treating critically ill patients.

In a flu pandemic, antiviral agents will be very important, particularly to limit spread in the early phases of the outbreak. Unregulated widespread use of antiviral drugs could cause drug-resistant strains to emerge and circulate, thus limiting drug effectiveness. Vaccines will be needed to provide long-term immunity. Each state and local community should have drug and vaccine distribution plans guided by federal recommendations. These plans should address:

> ➤ Antiviral stocks to treat patients in hospitals, clinics, nursing homes, alternate care facilities, and other locations.

> ➤ Antiviral stocks for postexposure prophylaxis (eg, direct contacts of infected casualties).

> ➤ Antiviral stocks for use in pre-exposure and postexposure prophylaxis (if recommended for health care workers, public safety workers, and others).

Pandemic plans need to be specific, practical, and practiced in tabletop and field exercises. State and local health authorities should review pandemic preparedness plans continually, including capacities and capabilities for disease surveillance, laboratory testing, and communication. Plans should include:

➤ Clear, effective, and coordinated risk communication, domestically and globally, before and during a pandemic. Credible spokespeople should be identified at all levels of government and within community organizations to deliver helpful, informative messages in a timely manner.

➤ Guidance to the private sector and critical infrastructure entities on their role(s) in the pandemic response, and consideration of what is necessary to maintain essential services and operations despite significant and sustained worker absenteeism.

➤ Guidance to individuals on infection control behaviors that should be adopted before a pandemic, and the specific actions they will need to take during a severe pandemic, such as self-isolation to protect others if individuals are exposed or infected.

4.11.2 Surveillance and Detection

Assessment of the rate of spread and outcome of a pandemic disease depends on effective and efficient public health surveillance systems. Physicians and other health professionals play an essential role in the detection of initial cases. If implemented early, identification and management of infected and exposed persons may help slow the spread of a communicable disease within the community.

Clinical awareness of the disease also benefits individual casualties, as rapid diagnosis and initiation of treatment can avert potentially severe complications. For influenza, detection may be complicated, however, by the lack of specific clinical findings and commercially available laboratory tests that can rapidly distinguish novel or pandemic influenza from seasonal influenza. In addition, neither the clinical characteristics of a novel or pandemic influenza virus strain, nor the groups at highest risk for complications, can necessarily be defined beforehand.

In a pandemic, physicians and other health care professionals will continue to provide essential clinical services. These include identifying and triaging cases, beginning an efficient and comprehensive diagnostic workup, initiating specific treatment and other supportive therapy, and anticipating clinical complications. In addition, health care professionals have an important role in working with public health authorities to promote community and individual measures that prevent or control the spread of the disease.

Early warning of a pandemic and the ability to closely track the spread of the outbreak is critical to being able to rapidly employ resources to contain the disease. Effective surveillance and detection systems will help save lives by allowing states and localities to activate pandemic response plans. To support situational awareness, both domestically and globally, efforts should be directed at:

➤ Working through global, federal, state, and local health authorities to ensure transparency, scientific cooperation, and rapid reporting of disease.

➤ Providing adequate and effective risk communication to the public.

➤ Supporting the development of proper scientific and epidemiologic expertise in affected regions to ensure early recognition of changes in outbreak patterns and trends.

➤ Supporting the development and sustainability of sufficient US and host nation laboratory capacity and diagnostic reagents, in affected regions and domestically, to provide rapid confirmation of suspected cases.

➤ Advancing mechanisms for "real-time" clinical surveillance in domestic acute care settings such as emergency departments, intensive care units, and laboratories, so that local, state, federal, and global health officials have continuous awareness of the profile of the illness in communities.

➤ Developing and deploying rapid diagnostics with greater sensitivity and reproducibility to allow onsite diagnosis of pandemic agents in the United States and abroad, in animals and in humans, to facilitate early warning, outbreak control, and targeting of therapy.

➤ Expanding domestic livestock and wildlife surveillance activities for screening and monitoring animals that may harbor viruses and other infectious agents with pandemic potential.

For influenza, surveillance includes documentation by virologic testing of patients who are hospitalized with pneumonia, acute respiratory distress syndrome, or other respiratory illness with no alternative diagnosis. Physicians should ask all patients with fever and upper respiratory tract symptoms about recent travel history, as well as monitor clinically for suspicious cases of the disease. Novel influenza viruses can be confirmed by reverse transcriptase polymerase chain reaction (RT-PCR) or virus isolation from tissue cell culture with subtyping. RT-PCR testing of novel influenza viruses is not performed by most hospital laboratories and is available at state public health laboratories and the CDC. Viral culture of specimens from suspected novel influenza cases should be attempted only in laboratories that meet the biocontainment conditions for Biosafety Level 3, with enhancements or higher.

4.11.3   Containment

The initial response to the emergence of an infectious agent that spreads easily among humans will focus on containing the disease at its source, if feasible, and preventing a pandemic. Once the agent spreads beyond the initial source of the outbreak, the focus of containment activities will be on individual- and population-based measures that can help slow transmission. *Containment* refers to the

WHO plan to define and contain the outbreak in specific geographic regions. This is an aggressive, proactive plan to isolate individuals and communities that are infected with the virus to help prevent further transmission.

A pandemic agent does not respect geographic or political borders. Efforts to limit entry into and egress from affected areas represent opportunities to control, or at least slow, the spread of infection. The interdependence between countries and communities, reflected by extensive international and domestic travel, makes it unlikely that strict movement restrictions could be imposed effectively. Even if not fully successful, containment decisions can help slow the spread of the disease, allowing additional time for implementation of further control measures.

In a pandemic, the WHO will work closely with the CDC and health authorities from other countries to monitor the situation and take necessary action to limit the spread of the disease. Federal, state, and local health authorities will monitor the situation closely in the United States and provide instructions for health professionals, citizens, and communities. Federal authorities will work with state and local health officials to encourage and assist communities, businesses, and organizations in preparing for a pandemic. Containment strategies aimed at controlling and slowing the spread of the disease might include measures that affect individuals (eg, isolation and monitoring of contacts) as well as measures that affect groups or entire communities (eg, cancellation of public gatherings). Evacuations will most likely have no meaningful effect on the spread of disease and probably will be counterproductive; they will merely move a group of people likely to require services and health care to another site that is already overburdened or soon to be overburdened.

Guided by epidemiologic data, state and local public health authorities will implement the most appropriate measures to maximize impact on disease transmission and minimize impact on individual freedom of movement. Federal health officials will provide assistance to states and localities as requested, including sharing experiences of others and providing advice on decision making as the situation evolves. Although states and localities have primary responsibility for public health matters within their borders, including isolation and quarantine, under the authority of Section 361 of the Public Health Service Act (42 USC 264), the HHS secretary may make and enforce regulations necessary to prevent the introduction, transmission, or spread of communicable diseases from foreign countries into the United States or from one state or possession into another.

Containment measures applied to individuals may have limited impact in preventing the transmission of a pandemic due to the short incubation period of the disease agent, the ability of people with asymptomatic infection to transmit the disease, and the possibility that early symptoms among infected people may be nonspecific, delaying recognition and implementation of containment. Nevertheless, with a less efficiently transmitted disease, isolation and quarantine may have great effectiveness, slowing disease spread, allowing time for targeted use of clinical interventions, and increasing time for vaccine production and implementation of other pandemic response activities. With widespread disease transmission, individual quarantine is less likely to have an impact and probably would not be feasible to implement. Community-based containment measures, such as closing schools or restricting public gatherings, and informing individuals about hand hygiene and cough etiquette, would be health priorities.

The most effective means of protecting a people is to prevent the pandemic from reaching the nation, as well as slowing or limiting the spread of the outbreak once infection arrives. Containment strategies toward these ends should:

➤ Encourage all levels of government, domestically and globally, to take appropriate and lawful action to contain an outbreak within the borders of their community, province, state, or nation.

➤ Use governmental authorities where appropriate to limit nonessential movement of people, goods, and services into and out of areas where an outbreak occurs. This includes the development of screening and monitoring mechanisms and agreements to appropriately control travel and shipping from affected regions if necessary to protect unaffected populations.

➤ Provide guidance to all levels of government on the range of options for infection control and containment, including those circumstances where social distancing measures, limitations on gatherings, or quarantine authority may be an appropriate public health intervention.

➤ Emphasize the roles and responsibilities of individuals in preventing the spread of an outbreak and the risk to others if infection control practices are not followed.

➤ Provide guidance for states, localities, and industry on best practices to prevent the spread of the pandemic agent in commercial, domestic, and wild animals.

➤ Rapidly share information on travelers who may be carriers of or who may have been exposed to the pandemic agent for the purposes of contact tracing and outbreak investigation.

➤ Implement mechanisms for active and passive surveillance during the outbreak, both within and beyond government borders.

4.11.4   Coordinated Communication and Information Sharing

Once health authorities have determined that sustained and efficient human-to-human spread of an infectious disease has occurred, a cascade of response mechanisms should be initiated, from the site of the documented transmission to locations around the globe. At this point, health agencies and health care facilities should be well beyond the planning stage and should have initiated many of the components of their pandemic response plans. Controlling a pandemic requires coordination among global, federal, state, and local authorities, with all of these authorities communicating to the public. Public health officials should provide specific and timely information to the health care community on diagnosing and treating the disease.

An infectious agent with pandemic potential represents a risk to populations everywhere. Success in controlling the outbreak depends on the availability of scarce resources and how these resources are distributed. During the pandemic alert period, the CDC will issue case definitions for human infections. Once these definitions have been developed, state and local health departments will be notified via the CDC Health Alert Network. Federal, state, and local health authorities also will consider implementation of containment strategies in coordination with CDC quarantine stations at US entry ports.

With the recent H1N1 flu pandemic, the CDC issued guidance and announcements to advise health professionals and the public on the best course of action by using television, radio, print, and the Internet. Local television and radio station news broadcasts and public service announcements regularly transmitted information about measures to put in place to control the spread of the disease, such as closing schools, cancelling sporting events, and postponing public gatherings. Health messages stressed the importance of prevention and personal hygiene as the most basic and important way to prevent the spread of the virus. Local health authorities worked closely with clinicians and community leaders to develop alternative health care facilities, dedicated community hotlines, and communication systems to advise local residents about the disease and treatment options.

4.11.5   Travel Restrictions

In a pandemic or other serious public health emergency, public health officials have authority to implement various measures to control the spread of the disease. These include travel advisories, border restrictions, and limitations of domestic and global travel. Restrictions on international travel might be necessary, particularly travel by air. Limiting or canceling travel by domestic residents and citizens from affected countries will depend on the properties of the disease that emerges. Voluntary limitations on travel, by which individuals decide to limit their own personal risk by canceling nonessential trips, also will limit disease spread.

Once a pandemic is under way, exit screening of travelers from affected areas (source control) is likely to be more efficient than entry screening to identify ill travelers. Early in a pandemic, this intervention may decrease disease introductions into a country. Later, however, as the pandemic spreads within a country, ongoing indigenous transmission will likely exceed new introductions and, therefore, federal authorities may modify or discontinue this strategy. Because some infected people will be in the incubation period, be infected but asymptomatic, or have mild symptoms, it will not be possible to identify and isolate all arriving infected or ill passengers and quarantine their fellow passengers. If a sick passenger is identified after leaving an airport, it might not be possible to identify everyone that the person contacted within the incubation period. If the pandemic begins in or spreads to the United States, health authorities will consider screening outbound travelers to decrease the risk of transmitting the disease to other countries. State and local health officials also may implement travel-related measures to slow disease spread within the United States.

4.11.6   Social Distancing

To prepare for a pandemic, one key public health message should be learned by everyone: "Limiting social contact helps save lives."

The pandemic agent spreads only through human-to-human contact. To prevent infection, public health authorities will require communities to follow "social distancing" rules. Being around others who may be sick increases the likelihood of getting the disease. Until an effective vaccine or treatment is available, limiting contact among people will be the main strategy for helping to contain the disease and to prevent others from getting sick. Experience with past flu pandemics has shown that limiting contact among people during the outbreak can help slow the spread of the virus and save lives.

Social distancing is an important disease prevention strategy in which a community imposes limitations on social (face-to-face) interactions to reduce exposure to and transmission of the disease. These limitations could include, but are not restricted to, facility closures, cancellation of public gatherings, and shutting down mass transportation. Parents and caregivers need to prepare for the closing of schools (public and private schools, as well as colleges and universities) and childcare programs. Employers and employees need to plan for possible changes in work schedules and business operations to limit social interaction to the greatest extent possible without disrupting essential services.

In a flu pandemic, most sick people will be asked to stay home and will be given instructions on how to take care of themselves. By staying home, they will be less likely to expose others to the disease. Sick people will be advised to avoid going to the hospital unless they have severe respiratory problems or other serious symptoms as defined by health authorities. During the pandemic, hospitals may have room to treat only the sickest casualties and those who have special medical needs. Family members also may be asked to stay home if a person in the household is sick. Infected family members could spread the virus to others.

4.11.7   Mass Prophylaxis and Care

In a serious pandemic, there is a real likelihood that health care systems, particularly hospitals, will be overwhelmed. The only method to mitigate such an impact is to have plans in place that effectively allocate scarce hospital-based resources among incoming casualties, based on casualty need, availability of resources, and anticipated outcomes. Health professionals need to remain connected with public health authorities to ensure proper treatment of confirmed ill casualties, in accordance with established CDC guidelines.

Hospital staff and ill casualties may have to accept a different level of care during a pandemic. For example, sick people may be asked to stay home or be treated at an alternate care facility; and nurse-to-bed ratios may be decreased, meaning that each nurse will be responsible for more occupied beds. Individual casualties might not immediately receive ideal treatment because of resource limitations and disease severity. In a pandemic, physicians and other health professionals will likely need to shift their practice from devoting more attention to the most critically ill to (1) helping those who are most likely to survive with the scarcity of resources available and (2) preventing others from being infected. This shift in medical decision making will come from a central public health authority and will be implemented in all health care facilities and hospital systems.

In any infectious disease outbreak, public health authorities are responsible for developing community strategies to prevent or limit the spread of the disease. These include the following:

➤ Issuing guidance for the diagnosis, care, and reporting of the sick. Health officials will provide guidelines for the distribution of scarce medical resources to those who need them most, and for the management of all exposed and infected people. Isolation of sick people may occur in the home or the health care setting, depending on the severity of the illness and/or the current capacity of the health care system to provide care. Consideration should be given to providing sufficient quantities of effective medications and ensuring that there is a feasible distribution of these medications to homebound persons.

➤ Distributing medications to large numbers of the population, including locations for mass vaccination and treatment clinics and staffing of such clinics. A basic part of pandemic planning is the need to establish dispensing sites for distributing antibiotics or providing vaccinations in various community settings. The number of sites should be scalable depending on the anticipated need. While planning includes identifying and training site volunteers and staff before an event, there should also be refresher and "just-in-time" training available before administering prophylaxis to the public. There are roles for both medical and nonmedical volunteers.

➤ Coordinating efforts to manage potentially large numbers of people who die from the disease and require mortuary and burial services. These services may become overextended, causing delays in or loss of funerals, which will increase the distress of families.

Early in a pandemic, a vaccine will either not be available or only be available in limited supply. Prescribed medications, such as antivirals, may be effective, but there will not be enough for everyone who wants a prescription. Public health officials will work to develop a national stockpile of drugs to help treat and control the spread of the disease and support the production and testing of possible vaccines, including finding reliable and quicker ways to make large quantities of vaccines and medications.

According to the HHS *Pandemic Influenza Plan*, when a person meets both the clinical and epidemiologic criteria for a suspected case of novel influenza A, health care personnel should initiate the following activities:[40]

➤ Implement infection control precautions, including respiratory hygiene/ cough etiquette. Casualties should be placed on droplet precautions for a minimum of 14 days, unless there is full resolution of illness or another cause has been identified before that period has elapsed. Health care personnel should wear surgical or procedure masks on entering casualty rooms, consistent with droplet precautions, as well as gloves and gowns when indicated for standard precautions. Ideally, casualties should be admitted to single rooms, and movement within the hospital should be limited to medically necessary purposes only.

➤ Notify local and state health departments. Report each patient who meets the clinical and epidemiologic criteria for a suspected case of novel influenza to the state or local health department as quickly as possible to facilitate initiation of public health measures. Designate one person as a point of contact to update public health authorities on the patient's clinical status.

➤ Obtain clinical specimens for novel influenza A virus testing, and notify the local and state health departments to arrange testing. Testing will likely be directed by public health authorities. Optimal specimens for detecting novel influenza virus infection may include nasopharyngeal swabs; nasal swabs, washes, or aspirates; throat swabs; and tracheal aspirates for intubated patients. Acute (within 7 days of illness onset) and convalescent (2-3 weeks after the acute specimen and at least 3 weeks after illness onset) serum specimens should be obtained. Serologic testing for novel influenza virus infection can be performed only at the CDC.

➤ Evaluate alternative diagnoses. An alternative diagnosis should be based only on laboratory tests with high positive predictive value (eg, blood culture, viral culture, pleural fluid culture, transthoracic aspirate culture). If an alternate cause is identified, the possibility of coinfection with a novel influenza virus may still be considered if there is a strong epidemiologic link to exposure to novel influenza.

➤ Decide on inpatient or outpatient management. The decision to hospitalize a sick person with suspected novel influenza will be based on the physician's clinical and risk assessments, and whether adequate precautions can be taken at home to prevent the potential spread of infection. Patients cared for at home should be separated from other household members as much as possible. All household members should carefully follow recommendations for hand and cough hygiene, and tissues used by the sick person should be placed in a bag and disposed of with other household waste. Although no studies have assessed the use of masks at home to decrease the spread of infection, use of surgical or procedure masks by casualties and caregivers during interactions may be of benefit. Separation of eating utensils for use by a person with influenza is not necessary, as long as they are washed with warm water and soap.

➤ Initiate antiviral treatment as soon as possible, even if laboratory results are not yet available. Clinical trials have shown that antiviral drugs can decrease the seasonal influenza duration by several days when initiated within 48 hours of illness onset. The clinical effectiveness of antiviral drugs for treatment of novel influenza remains unknown, but it is likely that the earlier treatment is initiated, the greater the benefit. During the pandemic alert period, available virus isolates from any case of novel influenza will be tested for resistance to currently licensed antiviral medications.

➤ Assist public health officials with identification of potentially exposed contacts. After consulting with state and local public health officials, clinicians might be asked to help identify people exposed to the person with suspected novel influenza (particularly health care workers). In general, people in close contact with the case-casualty at any time beginning one day before the onset of illness are considered at risk. Close contacts might include household and social contacts, family members, workplace or school contacts, travelers, and/or health care professionals.

<table><tr><td>Federal Pandemic Influenza Resources</td></tr></table>

➤ Information on pandemic influenza is available at http://www.pandemicflu.gov, the official US government website on this topic. State pandemic plans can be found at http://www.flu.gov/professional/states/index.html.

➤ The CDC website (http://www.cdc.gov/h1n1flu/) provides authoritative resources for health professionals and the public. The CDC also provides a public information hotline at 800-CDC-INFO (800-232-4636). The line is available in English and Spanish, 24 hours a day, 7 days a week. Questions also can be e-mailed to cdcinfo@cdc.gov.

4.12 MASS FATALITY MANAGEMENT[42,43]

Disasters and public health emergencies can be lethal and result in large numbers of fatalities, overwhelming local capabilities. In such situations, local and regional mass fatality response systems can effectively carry out the management of human remains and respond to the needs of survivors. Although mass fatality management falls under the jurisdiction of the local medical examiner, coroner, or similar medicolegal authority, health professionals can play a role in mass fatality planning and response activities.

Mass fatality events require extensive efforts to facilitate the identification process, establish the cause of death, and determine the circumstances surrounding the event.

Resources may be overwhelmed at local jurisdictions, and assistance is often needed at the state and federal level. Being prepared for large-scale disasters will ultimately give local and regional response systems the ability to effectively manage small-scale disasters that can potentially overwhelm an area.

Mass fatality events typically fall outside the health sector. In prolonged events, health professionals may assume responsibilities for handling the dead within the hospital or health care facility. Health care professionals have a primary obligation to protect and preserve the health of their patients, families, and communities, as well as themselves. In mass fatality events falling outside the non–health sector, the health professional forms part of the first responder team to manage the injured and provide immediate care.

Management of the fatally wounded is often overlooked yet is an important part of disaster preparedness. To respond effectively and understand how their actions can influence the process of managing the dead, health professionals require a fundamental, basic level of education and training in mass fatality management.

4.12.1   Overview of a Mass Fatality Event

The overall response to a mass fatality event can be divided into three phases:

➤ The initial phase begins when the first responder arrives at the scene. This individual is usually a police officer or firefighter who may become the initial incident commander (IC) of the event. The initial IC assesses the situation, activates the disaster plan, and coordinates the activities of first responders in a prioritized fashion.

➤ The second phase begins when the community disaster plan is activated, and the predetermined IC and other officials take their roles. Police and fire department personnel stabilize the scene, control environmental hazards, and assist with rescue efforts. Emergency medical service (EMS) personnel perform triage, provide immediate medical care, and transport survivors to nearby hospitals. A public information officer coordinates media information. Support services are established to assist the rescue workers and survivors. Additional resources and assistance are obtained as needed.

➤ The final phase is the resolution phase, which involves removal and transport of any human remains, coordination of morgue services, and continued family support. Typically, the local medical examiner or coroner (MEC) acts as IC to coordinate these activities. Other efforts occurring during the resolution phase are geared toward restoring the community to a normal level of functioning.

A mass casualty event also becomes a mass fatality event when local resources are overwhelmed and unable to manage the fatalities. The MEC is central to managing such an event and has several legal responsibilities:

➤ Take charge of bodies where death was the result of an emergency or disaster.

➤ Identify the dead, and perform an examination and autopsy as indicated.

➤ Determine and record cause, circumstances, and manner of death.

➤ Maintain custody of unclaimed bodies until they are turned over to the county for burial.

➤ Issue death certificates.

Management of a mass fatality event involves four primary operational components: search and recovery; morgue operations; family assistance; and federal assistance.

4.12.2   Search and Recovery

Search and recovery activities for mass fatality events usually involve locating and removing bodies, body parts, and personal effects. *Personal effects* refers to items carried by, or being transported with, an individual. All human remains should be treated with respect and dignity at all times and should be kept covered if possible. Search teams perform a systematic search of the disaster site, and aggressive efforts are made to safely rescue any potential survivors. All human remains and personal belongings should be identified and tagged with a unique number. If the human remains are scattered over an extensive area, a grid is useful to help document location, recreate the scene, and gather other information for the investigation. It is important to remember that every site should be treated as a crime scene unless otherwise indicated by the medical examiner or coroner (MEC).

Recovery begins after the search of a given area is complete. As long as there is no danger of further disintegration, human remains should not be moved from the scene before the arrival of the forensic expert in charge. If any dangers exist, the bodies should be moved immediately to a safe fatality collection point and secured from public view. Human remains are then transported to an established *identification center or temporary morgue*, where identification procedures are initiated. The location of the temporary morgue should be secluded, and any expectant (still living) casualties should *not* be in proximity to those already deceased.

4.12.3   Morgue Operations

The identification center or temporary morgue is divided into several different stations to record and provide information for eventual comparison to antemortem records. The information is used to confirm identification and facts surrounding a fatality. Ideally, human remains are assigned individual escorts during the process through each station to ensure that the remains are not mixed up with other remains, that documentation is complete, and that proper respect is paid to the remains at all times. Any form of identification (such as a driver's license) found in the vicinity of the remains may be useful information, but it does not confirm identification. Trauma from catastrophic disasters may result in significant distortion of facial features, and accurate identification uses an extensive process. The MEC can request assistance from experts in pathology, anthropology, dentistry, mortuary affairs, and search and recovery to assist with identification procedures.

Specific morgue activities include:

➤ Body cooling to prevent decomposition. A recommended temperature for human remains is 4°C, and freezing should be avoided. The use of Quicklime, Formal, or Zeolite may be required in disaster situations when cooling services are overwhelmed.

➤ Holding, visiting, and examination areas for crime scene investigations.

➤ Security to limit morgue access.

➤ Careful organized handling and labeling of remains and body parts.

➤ Meticulous record keeping and organization of morgue data and chain-of-custody procedures.

4.12.4   Family Assistance Centers (FACs)

A FAC should be carefully selected and established quickly in a site such as a hotel, conference center, school, or church. The location should be away from the actual scene, easily accessible to family members, and able to accommodate families coming from out of town. The area should be secured, limited to family members of the dead, and protected from the media. Family meetings should be conducted on an individual basis as soon as possible to collect antemortem information for use in the identification process. Regular briefings by the medical examiner/coroner or staff should take place to keep the families informed. Official identification of the deceased should be given to the families by the MEC in the presence of a grief counselor or appropriate religious support. Several resources should be on site to provide family assistance and support. The American Red Cross can assist with family support, transportation, housing, supplies, and volunteer coordination. Mental health professionals and clergy should be made available. Additional communication lines should be provided, and food service should be accessible.

Many misconceptions and concerns exist about the management of remains. Religious and social customs and population/community concerns should be included in the planning and response to any mass fatality event. FACs should adhere to social customs and norms in the community, with staffing to include:

➤ Community leaders.

➤ Mental health providers.

➤ Religious leaders.

➤ Local social support groups.

➤ Local Red Cross members.

➤ US Air Force urban search and rescue personnel.

➤ Local military personnel (if in proximity).

➤ Media in a separate "media space" to allow for more effective crisis communication.

➤ Police in a separate area to obtain antemortem information on the event from witnesses.

4.12.5   Federal Assistance

Federal resources may be requested to assist with state and local efforts in a mass fatality event. Within the National Response Framework, ESF-8 charges the HHS with the task of providing medical and public health assistance to state and local resources in response to mass casualty events. This includes coordination of the NDMS to provide medical assistance, casualty identification, and mortuary services. Disaster Mortuary Operational Response Teams (DMORTs) consist of forensic scientists (anthropologists, dentists, and pathologists), funeral directors, embalmers, medical records technicians, medicolegal investigators, and specialists in mass fatality management.

DMORT teams can be activated only for events that are declared disasters by the US President, and they support, not supplant, the local MEC. Other federal resources include the National Foundation of Mortuary Care (NFMC) and the Office of Armed Forces Medical Examiner (OAFME). The NFMC is a nonprofit organization that assists civil authorities with incident command and mortuary services during mass fatality incidents. It also recruits and trains DMORT members. The OAFME is required to investigate all federal and military crashes and deaths, and OAFME staff can respond to nonmilitary mass fatality incidents if a special request is made. The Federal Bureau of Investigation (FBI) may assist with the identification of remains and investigate criminal acts associated with terrorism.

The National Transportation Safety Board (NTSB) is charged with assisting the recovery of fatalities from aviation crashes as mandated by the Family Assistance Act of 1996. The identification process of these fatalities may remain under the jurisdiction of the local MEC.

4.12.6   Public Health Aspects of a Mass Fatality Event

Contrary to conventional thought, human remains are *not* public health menaces, and do not, in general, contribute to outbreaks of disease. However, remains that were infected antemortem may require different handling practices. Infectious agents that require precautions include:

➤ *Mycobacterium tuberculosis.*

➤ *Salmonella* species.

➤ *Vibrio cholerae.*

➤ Viral hemorrhagic fever viruses.

➤ Hepatitis B and C viruses.

➤ Influenza viruses.

➤ HIV (may survive 16 days in bodies).

➤ Prions (Creutzfeldt-Jakob disease).

Diseases caused by these agents, especially cholera, can lead to spread of disease and require special handling processes. However, outbreaks of disease attributable to human remains and dead animals that are uninfected with such illnesses are *not* expected.

Personal protection for mortuary workers can be adapted to the situation, but disposable clothing is best. Face masks are not particularly necessary and may hinder breathing, but many workers use them to decrease exposure to off-gassing fumes. Standard hygiene is sufficient. Hypochlorite solution for cleaning is adequate for most circumstances.

4.12.7   Mental Health Implications of a Mass Fatality Event

A mass fatality event challenges the coping skills of responders, hospital staff, relatives, and friends. Multidimensional support services and trained personnel can facilitate recovery. Local authorities should address the following issues:

➤ Unresolved grief at the scene.

➤ Timely and accurate communications from authorities that dispel fear.

➤ Dignity in death based on cultural norms and religious preferences.

➤ Early notification of death to survivors.

➤ Care and support to survivors.

➤ Final arrangements for the remains.

➤ Limited interviews with prepared statements for anticipated questions and without speculation.

4.12.8   Application of the DISASTER Paradigm to Mass Fatality Events

Preservation of life takes precedence over mass fatality management. The DISASTER paradigm offers a conceptual framework for effective mass fatality management.

Detection: An evaluation team consisting of fire or EMS personnel, the MEC, and a representative from the Incident Command Center should perform the following functions at the scene:

➤ Estimate the approximate number of fatalities involved.

➤ Identify the condition of the bodies (ie, burned, dismembered, entrapped).

➤ Assess any difficulty anticipated in the recovery of the bodies and the types of personnel and equipment needed (fire search and rescue, heavy equipment, HAZMAT team, personal protective equipment [PPE] for possible chemical, radiologic, or biologic hazards).

➤ Assess the location of the incident with regard to accessibility and transport issues for bodies.

➤ Select the temporary morgue or identification center location.

➤ Obtain additional personnel to assist with body identification, examination, and evidence collection.

Incident management: At the scene, the incident command team should work with the MEC to ensure:

➤ Identification of the dead.

➤ Location and resourcing of temporary morgues.

➤ Establishment of FACs.

Safety and security: Police and fire department personnel should secure the perimeter and control the environment for safety, as in any mass casualty incident. Only authorized individuals should be allowed within the perimeter. Family members of the dead should be referred to the FAC. Human remains should remain covered and out of public view as much as possible. Recovery efforts should not take place until it is deemed safe to do so. Search and rescue of the living trumps search and recovery of the dead. Every precaution must be taken to prevent injury to rescue and recovery workers.

Assess hazards: The MEC must have a sufficient number of people capable of functioning in a contaminated area. Universal precautions apply, and PPE should be provided. After assessing the overall scene and speaking with other incident managers (eg, fire and HAZMAT personnel), the MEC and search team leader should assess what the hazards are and what actions should be taken to mitigate them. Hazardous areas may include all human remains, chemical contamination, radiation exposure, and harmful animals.

With chemical or radiologic events, detailed information on agents, such as material safety data sheets (MSDS), and level of PPE required should be obtained from the IC at the scene. Appropriate decontamination solvents, safe handling procedures, and mechanisms for chemical monitoring should be determined. In such an incident, the MEC should be prepared to establish a preliminary morgue at the incident site to gather evidence from the remains before they undergo decontamination, which may result in evidence being lost. In the event of a terrorist incident involving chemical agents, an FBI HAZMAT technician, a law enforcement evidence collection technician, and a forensic odontologist should be included in the initial evaluation team.

Support: In a mass fatality event, an assessment should be made by the MEC, the IC, and the county emergency management director about the need for additional resources. When indicated, the county should declare a local emergency and call on state resources for assistance; the state in turn will petition for federal resources as needed. Several local organizations may have experience in mass fatality response and should be included in any mass fatality situation. Contact information for additional resources should be included in community mass fatality response plans.

Potential Contacts in a Mass Fatality Event

Local

➤ County medical examiners and staff.

➤ Local urban search and rescue group.

➤ Refrigerated truck service.

➤ Utility services (water, electricity).

➤ Food services.

➤ Mental health and religious support.

➤ Local Red Cross, to assist with establishing FACs.

➤ National Guard or Army Reserve unit.

➤ University or college with forensic anthropology expertise.

➤ Site support (custodial and site maintenance).

➤ Communications and information systems support.

➤ Media, to disseminate information.

State

➤ Division of Emergency Management.

➤ Department of Public Safety (crime laboratory).

➤ State Health Laboratory, to coordinate with CDC.

➤ State Board of Funeral Directors and Embalmers.

➤ State Funeral Directors Association.

➤ Dental association disaster team.

National

➤ National Disaster Medical System (DMORT teams).

➤ Department of Justice: FBI.

➤ Department of Defense: Mortuary Services.

➤ NTSB.

➤ Bureau of Alcohol, Tobacco, Firearms and Explosives.

➤ CDC.

➤ National Funeral Directors Association.

Volunteer

➤ American Red Cross.

➤ Salvation Army.

➤ Critical Incident Stress Debriefing Network.

Triage and treatment: The triage officer at the disaster scene should inform the MEC of casualties triaged into the "expectant" category as a way to anticipate emerging fatalities. If decontamination is required, a preliminary morgue should be established at the site of decontamination, as some evidence may be lost during the decontamination process. Remains should then be brought to the temporary morgue or identification center where identification procedures are initiated:

➤ In-processing: establishes chain-of-custody documents and starts tracking of human remains.

➤ Photography and full-body radiology: photographs remains as they are received; full-body radiology may be done to locate objects or personnel effects embedded within the remains.

➤ Personal effects station: collects, documents, and stores clothing and other personal items.

➤ Fingerprinting.

➤ Pathology section: performs autopsy to confirm the manner of death and obtain samples for laboratory tests and DNA analysis as indicated by protocol.

➤ Forensic logistics/hemogenetics section: performs dental tests, somatometry (measurement), blood typing, HLA and DNA profiling.

➤ Dental section: processes antemortem and postmortem dental records for identification.

➤ Physical anthropology: provides information regarding age, sex, racial origin, and skeletal abnormalities to assist with identification.

➤ Mortuary science section: prepares remains for release; performs embalming.

Evacuation and recovery: After a body has been identified, the family should be informed as soon as possible by the MEC or designee. Mental health, religious support, and social services should be available. Cremation should not take place in a mass fatality temporary morgue or identification center. The body should be released from the morgue after identification is confirmed and moved to a place designated by the family. Personal effects are important for families and should be returned to them as soon as possible when requested. Unidentifiable bodies can be embalmed and stored pending further investigation.

4.13 ENHANCING COMMUNITY RESILIENCE FOR DISASTER RECOVERY

Prevention, preparedness, and wellness strategies are essential to help individuals and communities develop the resiliency and the coping skills to deal with health challenges. Evidence supports various protective factors that may ameliorate risks to overall health: immunizations, exercise, good nutrition, adequate rest, healthy human interactions, and support from peers. Casualty and employee assistance, substance use intervention programs, access to peer and professional counseling, and social inclusion enhance health and well-being. Those who take the time to prepare and practice a personal, family, and workplace disaster plan are more likely to cope with the physical and emotional trauma associated with disasters.

In 2007, Homeland Security Presidential Directive 21 (HSPD-21) identified community resilience as one of the "four most critical components of public health and medical preparedness," along with biosurveillance, countermeasure distribution, and mass casualty care.[44] The directive also recognized "the important roles of individuals, families, and communities," and advocated for health curricula and training to "enhance private citizen opportunities for contributions to local, regional, and national preparedness and response." Building community resilience requires a holistic approach that takes into consideration appropriate developmental, cultural, and linguistic strategies.[45–47]

Various "prevention, preparedness, and wellness" strategies can be integrated through an analysis of personal and community hazards, vulnerabilities, and risks. Health professionals can use educational and informational resources to:

➤ Prevent the occurrence of death, injury, or illness in a disaster or public health emergency.

➤ Mitigate the medical and mental health consequences of a disaster or public health emergency.

➤ Minimize the effects of injury, disease, and disability among those with pre-existing health conditions in a disaster or public health emergency.

➤ Enhance personal and community capacity to prepare for, respond to, and cope with disasters and public health emergencies.

Reduction of injury, disease, and disability in the United States requires communities, families, and policymakers to advocate for a coherent and effective prevention, preparedness, and wellness strategy, recognize its importance in public health policy, and work toward making it a priority in this country.

4.14 AFTER-ACTION REPORTING

Responders may be requested to participate in a debriefing ("hot wash") to discuss the strengths, weaknesses, and opportunities for improvement related to operational responses. Findings of the debriefing are captured in a report called the after-action report (AAR). The AAR is an analysis that summarizes the strengths and identifies the major problems and issues of the disaster operation. It denotes the lessons learned from the response and deployment. In addition, the report includes recommendation to improve future operations. A supporting document is the Improvement Plan (IP). The IP indicates the steps for accomplishing the recommended changes. A volunteer who is deployed federally is not likely to be tasked with writing an AAR. However, it is helpful to learn about the components and keep these in mind as one records thoughts on deployment experience.

A thorough post-event analysis with an AAR report is imperative to determine the overall successes and shortfalls of the disaster casualty management system. The goal of after-action reporting is to evaluate performance, find problems, describe how challenges were overcome, and provide a lessons-learned venue for those who may encounter a similar situation in the future. An important part of the AAR is a performance assessment. How well did the plan work? Were the assumptions in the disaster plan accurate? How good was the training? Did the ICS work as exercised? What improvements can be made? What lessons were learned? The questions are many, yet the opportunity they present for learning about the overall response to improve future responses is worth the effort. All information derived from this process should be combined in an AAR so that others can view the information and learn from the experience. By participating directly in the review process, responders can learn what worked and what did not, which provides an opportunity for professional growth and improvement.

After action reviews should be conducted as soon as practical after the event and again several days later after the experiences have been digested. The timeframe for the debriefing is after stabilization of incident, but before key staff members are demobilized. By revisiting the event, beginning with the disaster plan, and studying what went right and where improvement opportunities exist, emergency planners and managers can be better prepared for future events. These reviews and reports provide the basis for changing response plans and developing table top and full-field exercises to test the assumptions and recommendations made in AARs. After appropriate evaluation and refinement, the assumptions and recommendations should become part of standard practices and perhaps even best practices.

NIMS includes resources for post-incident analysis, critique, and lessons learned. Having a consistent approach for all phases of disaster management makes collaborative learning and information-sharing among multiple agencies and organizations a real possibility and a staple in strengthening national disaster preparedness.

Key Components of an After-Action Report (AAR)[48]

Executive Summary (describe briefly contents of report: overview of event, major strengths identified, areas requiring improvement)

Section I: Overview (usually bullet points rather than paragraph format)

➤ Event details (type of hazard, start/end date, duration, location, single/multi-jurisdiction involvement.

➤ Participating organizations (international, federal, state, local, tribal, non-government).

➤ Number of participants (total players, controllers, evaluators, observers).

Section 2: Summary (main objectives, what actually happened, strengths and recommendations for improvement)

Section 3: Analysis of Capabilities (review the performance of capabilities, activities, and tasks related to mitigation, preparedness, response, and recovery)

Section 4: Conclusion

➤ Major lessons learned.

➤ Lessons learned through response/recover phases.

➤ Lessons learned from other organizations.

➤ Summary of what improvement processes/steps are needed to refine plans, policies, procedures, and training for this type of incident.

Supporting Document: Improvement Plan (often presented in table format)

➤ List each recommendation separately.

➤ Denote capability related to each recommendation.

➤ State organization and/or who is responsible to complete recommendation.

➤ Provide proposed timeframe for completion.

➤ List actual completion date.

Helpful hints for writing an AAR:

➤ Use legible script in handwriting.

➤ Use plain English.

➤ Avoid abbreviations and jargon.

➤ Be clear and concise.

➤ Include known facts and not rumors or hear-say information.

➤ Submit in timely manner.

➤ Share with relevant parties.

4.15 SUMMARY

Integration of all medical and public health assets in the community is a necessary step toward increasing response capacity and capability. This requires that disparate local health and medical organizations plan collaboratively for a coordinated, community-wide emergency response. In a large-scale disaster or public health emergency, health response organizations will be expected to work together, share response plans, and have a commonly understood framework for coordination under the urgency and uncertainty of a rapidly evolving incident. A framework for such coordination, such as a NIMS-compliant HEOC, will integrate hospital administrators, physicians, EMS, community health clinics, pharmacists, and other caregivers with the public health and emergency management agencies.

Functions of the public health system include situational awareness, surveillance, population-based triage, risk communication, mass care, mass prophylaxis, and mass fatality management. Across government levels (federal, state, and local), the public health system helps to ensure appropriate care for all ages and populations through health monitoring, disease surveillance, and laboratory sciences. Additionally, the public health system acts as the expert system for tracking, predicting, and developing response tactics to disease outbreaks or other health threats. The public health system has a role in communicating prevention strategies as well as information about self-care and shelter-in-place strategies during a crisis. In an emergency, the public may be advised to seek care or reassurance in alternate settings so that hospitals and emergency care facilities can focus resources on those who need them most. The DISASTER paradigm is a useful guide for effective mass fatality response. Ultimately, community recovery depends on the reservoir of community resilience. Ready clinical, public health, and emergency management professionals enable community resilience.

10 Questions to Define Professional Readiness for Disaster Response

What is your role in your organization's disaster plan?

How is your organization's disaster plan activated?

How are you notified of disaster plan activation?

Where do you report when your organization's disaster plan is activated?

Where is your organization's emergency operations center located?

How does your organization fit into your community's disaster plan?

What mutual aid agreements does your organization have with other organizations?

Are you registered as a volunteer in the Emergency System for Advance Registration of Volunteer Health Professionals (ESAR-VHP) and/or with professional societies for disaster response?

Is your license linked to a state registry of volunteer disaster responders?

Have you considered joining the Medical Reserve Corps (MRC) or a Disaster Medical Assistance Team (DMAT)?

REFERENCES

1. Subbarao I, Lyznicki JM, Hsu EB, et al. A consensus-based educational framework and competency set for the discipline of disaster medicine and public health preparedness. *Disaster Med Public Health Prep.* 2008;2:57–68.

2. The White House. *The Federal Response to Hurricane Katrina: Lessons Learned.* Washington, DC: US Government Printing Office; 2006. http://georgewbush-whitehouse.archives.gov/reports/katrina-lessons-learned/. Accessed March 27, 2011.

3. Select Bipartisan Committee to Investigate the Preparation for and Response to Hurricane Katrina, US House of Representatives. *A Failure of Initiative.* Washington, DC: US Government Printing Office; 2006. http://www.katrina.house.gov/. Accessed March 27, 2011.

4. Committee on Homeland Security and Governmental Affairs, US Senate. *Hurricane Katrina: A Nation Still Unprepared.* Washington, DC: US Government Printing Office; 2006. http://www.gpoaccess.gov/serialset/creports/katrinanation.html. Accessed March 27, 2011.

5. US Government Accountability Office. *Catastrophic Disasters: Enhanced Leadership, Capabilities, and Accountability Controls Will Improve the Effectiveness of the Nation's Preparedness, Response, and Recovery System.* GAO-06-618. Washington, DC: General Accountability Office; 2006. http://www.gao.gov/products/GAO-06-618. Accessed March 27, 2011.

6. Aldrich N, Benson WF. Disaster preparedness and the chronic disease needs of vulnerable older adults [serial online]. *Preventing Chronic Dis.* 2006;3:1–7. http://www.cdc.gov/Pcd/issues/2008/jan/pdf/07_0135.pdf. Accessed March 27, 2011.

7. Sharma AJ, Weiss EC, Young SL, et al. Chronic disease and related conditions at emergency treatment facilities in the New Orleans area after Hurricane Katrina. *Disaster Med Public Health Prep.* 2008;2:27–32.

8. Brodie M, Weltzien E, Altman D, Blendon RJ, Benson JM. Experiences of Hurricane Katrina evacuees in Houston shelters: implications for future planning. *Am J Public Health.* 2006;96:1402–1408.

9. Hurricane Katrina Community Advisory Group, Kessler RC. Hurricane Katrina's impact on the care of survivors with chronic medical conditions. *J Gen Intern Med.* 2007;22:1225–1230.

10. Stephens KU, Grew D, Chin K, et al. Excess mortality in the aftermath of Hurricane Katrina: a preliminary report. *Disaster Med Public Health Prep.* 2007;1:15–20.

11. Jhung MA, Shehab N, Rohr-Allegrini C, Pollack DA, Sanchez R, Guerra F, et al. Chronic disease and disasters: medication demands of Hurricane Katrina evacuees. *Am J Prev Med.* 2007;33:207–210.

12. Greenough GP, Lappi MD, Hsu EB, et al. Burden of disease and health status among Hurricane-Katrina-displaced persons in shelters: a population-based cluster sample. *Ann Emerg Med.* 2008;51:426–432.

13. Tam VC, Knowles SR, Cornish PL, Fine N, Marchesano R, Etchells EE. Frequency, type and clinical importance of medical history errors at admission to hospital: a systemic review. *CMAJ.* 2005;173:510–515.

14. Canino G, Bravo, M, Rubio-Stipec M, et al. The impact of disaster on mental health: prospective and retrospective analyses. *Int J Ment Health.* 1990;19:51–69.

15. Madakasira S, O'Brien KF. Acute posttraumatic stress disorder in victims of a natural disaster. *J Nerv Ment Dis.* 1987;175:286–290.

16. Ranasinghe PD, Levy BR. Prevalence of and sex disparities in posttraumatic stress disorder in an internally displaced Sri Lankan population six months after the Tsunami. *Disaster Med Public Health Prep.* 2007;1:34–43.

17. Galea S, Brewin CR, Gruber M, Jones RT, King DW, King LA, et al. Exposure to hurricane-related stressors and mental illness after Hurricane Katrina. *Arch Gen Psychiatry.* 2007;64:1427–1434.

18. Centers for Disease Control and Prevention. *Public Health's Infrastructure: A Status Report to the U.S. Senate Appropriations Committee.* Washington, DC: US Government Printing Office; 2001. http://www.uic.edu/sph/prepare/courses/ph410/resources/phinfrastructure.pdf. Accessed March 27, 2011.

19. Lister SA. *An Overview of the U.S. Public Health System in the Context of Emergency Preparedness.* Order Code RL31719. Washington, DC: Congressional Research Service; 2005. http://www.fas.org/sgp/crs/homesec/RL31719.pdf. Accessed March 27, 2011.

20. Heyman DL, ed. *Control of Communicable Diseases Manual.* 19th ed. Washington, DC: American Public Health Association; 2008.

21. Landesman LY. *Public Health Management of Disasters: The Practice Guide.* 2nd ed. Washington, DC: American Public Health Association; 2005.

22. Centers for Disease Control and Prevention. *Public Health Emergency Response Guide for State, Local and Tribal Public Health Directors*. Version 1.0. http://www.emergency.cdc.gov/planning/pdf/cdcresponseguide.pdf. Accessed March 27, 2011.

23. Pan American Health Organization (PAHO). *Natural Disasters: Protecting the Public's Health*. Scientific Publication No. 575. Washington, DC: PAHO; 2000.

24. Noji EK, ed. *The Public Health Consequences of Disasters*. New York, NY: Oxford University Press; 1997.

25. Barbera J, McIntyre A. *Medical Surge Capacity and Capability: A Management System for Integrating Medical and Health Resources During Large-Scale Emergencies*. 2nd ed. Alexandria, VA: CNA Corp; 2007. http://www.ncdhhs.gov/dhsr/EMS/aspr/pdf/mscc.pdf. Accessed March 27, 2011.

26. Burkle FM, Hsu EB, Loehr M, et al. Definitions and functions of health unified command and emergency operations centers for large-scale bioevent disasters within the existing ICS. *Disaster Med Public Health Prep*. 2007;1:135–141.

27. Burkle FM. Population-based triage management in response to surge-capacity requirements during a large-scale bioevent disaster. *Acad Emerg Med*. 2006;13:118–129.

28. Bostick NA, Subbarao I, Burkle FM Jr, Hsu EB, Armstrong JH, James JJ. Disaster triage systems for large-scale catastrophic events. *Disaster Med Public Health Prep*. 2008;2 (suppl 1):S35–S39.

29. HIPAA Privacy Rule and Public Health: Guidance from the Centers for Disease Control and Prevention and the U.S. Department of Health and Human Services. *MMWR*. 2003;52;1–12. http://www.cdc.gov/mmwr/preview/mmwrhtml/m2e411a1.htm. Accessed March 27, 2011.

30. Department of Health and Human Services. HIPAA Frequent Questions: Is the HIPAA Privacy Rule Suspended in a National of Public Health Emergency? http://www.hhs.gov/hipaafaq/providers/hipaa-1068.html. Accessed March 27, 2011.

31. US Department of Health and Human Services. *Communicating in a Crisis: Risk Communication Guidelines for Public Officials*. Washington, DC: Department of Health and Human Services; 2002. http://www.hhs.gov/od/documents/RiskCommunication.pdf. Accessed March 27, 2011.

32. Association of Public Health Laboratories. Core functions and capabilities of state public health laboratories. *MMWR*. 2002;51(RR14):1–8. http://www.cdc.gov/mmwr/preview/mmwrhtml/rr5114a1.htm. Accessed March 27, 2011.

33. Centers for Disease Control and Prevention. *The Laboratory Response Network*. http://www.bt.cdc.gov/lrn. Accessed March 27, 2011.

34. Kanter RK, Andrake JS, Boeing NM, et al. Developing consensus on appropriate standards of disaster care for children. *Disaster Med Public Health Prep*. 2009;3:27–32.

35. Kanter RK, Cooper A. Mass critical care: pediatric considerations in extending and rationing care in public health emergencies. *Disaster Med Public Health Prep*. 2009;3:S166.

36. *National Commission on Children and Disasters. 2010 Report to the President and Congress*. AHRQ Publication No. 10-M037. Rockville, MD. Agency for Healthcare Research and Quality; 2010. http://www.ahrq.gov/prep/nccdreport/nccdreport.pdf. Accessed March 27, 2011.

37. Arrieta MI, Foreman RD, Crook ED, Icenogle ML. Providing continuity of care for chronic disease in the aftermath of Katrina: from field experience to policy recommendations. *Disaster Med Public Health Prep*. 2009;3:174–182.

38. Federal Emergency Management Agency (FEMA). *Guidance on Planning for Integration of Functional Needs Support Services in General Population Shelters*. Washington, DC: US Government Printing Office; 2010. http://www.fema.gov/pdf/about/odic/fnss_guidance.pdf. Accessed March 27, 2011.

39. Knobler SL, Mack A, Mahmoud A, Lemon SM, eds. *The Threat of Pandemic Influenza: Are We Ready? A Workshop Report.* Washington, DC: National Academies Press; 2005.

40. US Department of Health and Human Services. *Pandemic Influenza Plan.* Washington, DC: US Government Printing Office; 2005. http://www.hhs.gov/pandemicflu/plan/pdf/HHSPandemicInfluenzaPlan.pdf. Accessed March 27, 2011.

41. World Health Organization (WHO). *Pandemic Influenza Preparedness and Response: A WHO Guidance Document.* Geneva, Switzerland: WHO; 2009. http://www.who.int/csr/disease/influenza/PIPGuidance09.pdf. Accessed March 27, 2011.

42. World Health Organization (WHO). *Management of Dead Bodies in Disaster Situations.* Disaster Manuals and Guidelines Series No. 5. Washington, DC: WHO and Pan American Health Organization; 2004. http://www.paho.org/english/dd/ped/DeadBodiesBook.pdf. Accessed March 27, 2011.

43. Centers for Disease Control and Prevention. *Interim Health Recommendations for Workers Who Handle Human Remains After a Disaster.* http://www.emergency.cdc.gov/disasters/handleremains.asp. Accessed March 27, 2011.

44. Homeland Security Presidential Directive 21 (HSPD-21). *Public Health and Medical Preparedness.* Washington, DC: The White House; 2007. http://www.fas.org/irp/offdocs/nspd/hspd-21.htm. Accessed March 27, 2011.

45. Norris FH, Stevens SP, Pfefferbaum B, Wyche KF, Pfefferbaum RL. Community resilience as a metaphor, theory, set of capacities, and strategy for disaster readiness. *Am J Community Psychology.* 2007;41:127–150.

46. Gurwitch RH, Pfefferbaum B, Montgomery JM, Klomp RW, Reissman DB. *Building Community Resilience for Children and Families.* Oklahoma City: Terrorism and Disaster Center, University of Oklahoma Health Sciences Center; 2007. http://www.oumedicine.com/Workfiles/College%20of%20Medicine/AD-Psychiatry/CR_guidebook.pdf. Accessed March 27, 2011.

47. US Department of Health and Human Services (HHS). *National Health Security Strategy of the United States of America.* Washington, DC: HHS;2009. http://www.phe.gov/Preparedness/planning/authority/nhss/Pages/default.aspx. Accessed March 27, 2011.

48. Office of the Civilian Volunteer Medical Reserve Corps. *Preparing For A Federal Deployment.* Fort Lauderdale: QuickSeries Publishing; 2010.

APPENDIX: EMERGENCY SUPPORT FUNCTION 8 (ESF-8), PUBLIC HEALTH AND MEDICAL SERVICES

1. Purpose: ESF-8 enables coordinated federal assistance to supplement state, tribal, and local resources in response to a potential or actual public health and medical disaster, such as a biologic event, and to a natural disaster. It includes the behavioral health needs of casualties and responders, medical response for ongoing health needs, and animal health.

2. The primary agency is the Department of Health and Human Services (HHS).

3. Actions include:

    a. Public health and medical needs assessment

    b. Public health surveillance

    c. Medical care personnel deployment

    d. Medical equipment and supplies distribution

    e. Patient evacuation and care

    f. Safety and security

    g. Blood, organs, and tissues

    h. Behavioral health care

    i. Public health and medical information

    j. Vector control

    k. Public health aspects of potable water, wastewater, and sewage

    l. Mass fatality management

    m. Veterinary medical support

4. Specialized resources and capabilities include:

    a. National Disaster Medical System (NDMS)

        i. Disaster Medical Assistance Teams (DMATs)

            ➤ General.

            ➤ Specialized (burn, pediatric, crush medicine, international).

        ii. National Medical Response Teams (NMRTs)

        iii. Disaster Mortuary Operational Response Teams (DMORTs)

        iv. Family Assistance Center (FAC) Teams

        v. Mental Health Teams

        vi. National Veterinary Response Teams (NVRTs)

b. Strategic National Stockpile (SNS)

c. Public Health Service Commissioned Corps

d. Incident Response Coordination Team (IRCT)

e. Applied Public Health Team (APHT): "public health department in a box"

f. Mental Health Teams (MHTs)

g. US Public Health Service Rapid Deployment Force (RDF)

5. Concept of operations:

a. In accordance with the Robert T. Stafford Act for Disaster Relief and Emergency Assistance (http://www.fpc.state.gov/documents/organization/53688.pdf; 1988), the governor of the involved state must make a disaster declaration before requesting aid. The President then declares a disaster and directs the Secretary of Health and Human Services to activate ESF-8. Under the Pandemic and All Hazards Preparedness Act (PAHPA; 2006), ESF-8 is the responsibility of the Assistant Secretary for Preparedness and Response (ASPR).

b. After deployment, teams conduct a risk analysis and determine the capabilities required to meet the mission objective. Public health and medical assistance is provided through state, tribal, and local medical and public health officials.

CHAPTER FIVE

Legal and Ethical Issues in Disasters

Matthew Wynia, MD, MPH

5.1 PURPOSE

This chapter discusses the legal and ethical frameworks for effective disaster planning and response.

5.2 LEARNING OBJECTIVES

After completing this chapter, readers will be able to:

➤ Describe the general legal and regulatory framework for disaster response.

➤ Discuss the three core ethical issues common in disaster planning and response (3 R's: responsibilities, restrictions, and rationing).

➤ Explain standards of care in disasters.

5.3 DISASTER MEDICINE AND PUBLIC HEALTH PREPAREDNESS COMPETENCIES ADDRESSED[1]

➤ Apply moral and ethical principles and policies to address individual and community health needs in a disaster. This includes understanding of the professional duty to treat, the right to protect personal safety in a disaster, and other responsibilities and rights of health care professionals in a disaster or public health emergency. (7.1.2)

➤ Apply legal principles, policies, and practices to address individual and community health needs in a disaster. This includes understanding of liability, worker protection and compensation, licensure, privacy, quarantine laws, and other legal issues to enable and encourage health care professionals to participate in disaster response and maintain the highest possible standards of care under extreme conditions. (7.2.2)

5.4 INTRODUCTION

[Dr Rieux] knew that the tale he had to tell . . . could be only the record of what had to be done, and what assuredly would have to be done again in the never ending fight against terror and its relentless onslaughts, despite their personal afflictions, by all who, while unable to be saints but refusing to bow down to pestilences, strive their utmost to be healers.[2]

Albert Camus, *The Plague*

In 2003, an outbreak of a novel coronavirus, causing severe acute respiratory syndrome (SARS), infected approximately 8400 people worldwide. The epidemic caused 813 deaths and billions of dollars in worldwide economic damage.[3] In Toronto, 45% of probable or suspect cases were among health care professionals.[4] In every affected nation, health care professionals had to choose between providing care and staying at home, crystallizing an ethical challenge.[5]

In October 2005, in the face of a potential avian flu pandemic, President George W. Bush declared that "the best way to deal with a pandemic is to isolate it and keep it isolated in the region in which it begins" and then invoked the possibility of using military force to do so.[6] Public health experts subsequently conveyed that influenza is not amenable to quarantine, since infected individuals are contagious before they know they are infected, and contemporary travel patterns create very rapid dispersal. Yet isolation and quarantine are age-old methods to mitigate infectious epidemics, with appeal on scientific, intuitive, and political grounds. When they are used, it is more often health care professionals than the military who must interact directly with the people involved and explain why their liberty is being restricted.

In 2001, mailed anthrax spores killed five, sickened 17, and caused hundreds of thousands of Americans to take antibiotics or get a prescription "just in case." Prescriptions for ciprofloxacin rose by approximately 160,000 in October 2001, and those for doxycycline rose by 216,000 in October and November.[7] Health care professionals faced with anxious and sometimes angry patients had to determine whom to provide with antibiotics when it appeared that acute shortages would arise. Anxiety about "white powder" seen anywhere led to a surge in testing by state public health laboratories to rule out anthrax.

These examples provide brief illustrations of the types of ethical and legal issues faced by health care professionals in public health emergencies. While a very broad array of ethical issues can arise,[8–10] for health care professionals, three issues are especially common and relevant:

1. Health care professionals have a shared responsibility to provide care during disasters, even when doing so might pose some risk to their own safety.[11] Understanding this "duty to treat," its limits, and related professional responsibilities associated with preparedness and recovery, are keys to effective disaster response.[12,13]

2. Health care professionals are often caught in decision-making and implementation dilemmas related to restricting individual liberty to protect the larger public's health. Determining when, how, and whom to subject to isolation or quarantine, for example, entails scientific understanding as well as recognition of important social, psychological, community, and legal dynamics.[14]

3. While many resource allocation decisions are made by organizations, such as state agencies or hospitals, individual health care professionals are involved in implementing plans to fairly allocate scarce resources when the need outstrips their availability.[15] In disasters, health care professionals have faced the need to alter dramatically the level of care they provide relative to what they might have provided under normal circumstances. There is no ethically simple or comfortable response to such dilemmas, yet they can arise and should be anticipated in public dialogue and addressed in training and planning.[16]

5.5   LEGAL BACKGROUND

Ethics and the law are related, but distinct, and some background regarding US Constitutional law is important for understanding the role of health care professionals in public health emergencies. The US Constitution and subsequent amendments assert a number of important individual rights. Of particular importance to disaster planning and response are the rights to due process and equal protection under the law guaranteed by the 5th and 14th Amendments. As a result, only under specific conditions may the individual liberties of US citizens be restricted by the government. There must be a compelling interest, such as keeping dangerous people away from society or preventing a danger from spreading (eg, an epidemic). The proposed intervention must be well targeted. It must use the least restrictive means necessary, and due process (ie, some form of appeal or other mechanism to ensure the legitimacy of the action) must be available to those whose liberty is being limited.

In addition, the US Constitution lays out specific roles for the federal and state governments. The federal government is charged with regulating interstate commerce, providing for the national defense, and promoting the public welfare. All other powers of governing, including almost all authority directly pertaining to public health law and so-called police powers, are reserved for the states.

Police powers enable a state to protect public health and welfare, and they include public health emergency powers.

Public health emergency powers include surveillance, reporting, epidemiologic investigation, property seizure, voluntary or mandatory vaccination, isolation, social distancing (eg, closure of schools, public buildings, and public gathering places such as shopping malls), and evacuation of facilities or areas. While the specific process and powers can vary by state, the general process is initiated by the governor, who declares a public health emergency; this permits public health authorities to use emergency powers. The governor can mobilize the state National Guard as well.

In addressing the disaster, the governor can also ask for federal assistance, which can be provided by the Secretary of Health and Human Services and by the president. Short of anarchy, the federal government cannot intervene without state invitation. This follows a long tradition of states' rights in the United States. The Insurrection Act (1807), from the age of Thomas Jefferson, limits use of federal forces within states, and the Posse Comitatus Act (1878), passed during Reconstruction, prohibits use of federal troops for law enforcement. The Stafford Act (1988) defines the process for federal intervention in disasters and requires the governor to ask for assistance first. Following this request, the president can declare a disaster, and federal agencies such as the Federal Emergency Management Agency (FEMA) can respond.

FIGURE 5-1
Government Pillars of
Disaster Response

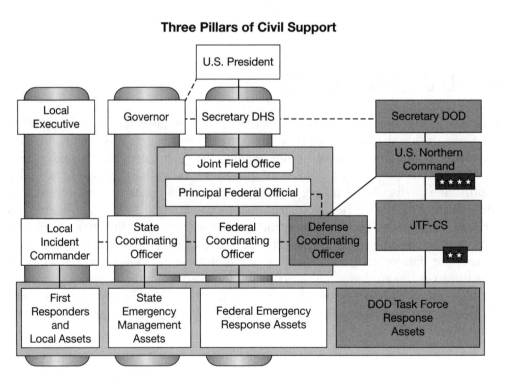

Three Pillars of Civil Support

DHS, Department of Homeland Security; DOD, Department of Defense; JTF-CS, Joint Task Force–Civil Support. A joint task force includes more than one branch of the armed forces. Source: JTF Command Briefing, 2005.

Figure 5-1 shows several "pillars" of disaster response, including the possible assistance of the US military. The military can become involved, on request of civil authorities, through coordination between the Secretary of Homeland Security and the Secretary of the Department of Defense. After 9/11, the federal government recognized that the US military was structured to respond to disasters around the globe *except* in North America. Thus was born the US Northern Command to cover security requirements for North America.

5.6 PROFESSIONAL RESPONSIBILITIES

Every man that undertakes to be of a profession or takes upon himself an office must take all parts of it, the good and the evil, the pleasure and the pain, the profit and the inconveniences all together and not pick and choose; for Ministers must preach, Captains must fight, and Physicians attend upon the sick.[17]

William Boghurst, Apothecary, Great Plague of London, 1666

While the obligation to continue caring for patients in the face of personal risk is not found in the Hippocratic oath (though a duty to care for the poor is there), it has been a central tenet of American medical professionalism since 1847.[11] American physicians wrote in the first Code of Ethics of the American Medical Association (AMA), "When pestilence prevails, it is [the professionals'] duty to face the danger, and to continue their labors for the alleviation of suffering, even at the jeopardy of their own lives."[18]

The AMA Code was written specifically to create *reciprocal obligations* between medicine and society, and as such, it made medicine's prerogatives and social standing contingent on physicians continuing to provide care when epidemics occurred.[11] Since epidemics at the time were common, this promise was remarkable and very powerful. Between 1920 and 1940, 10% of medical students developed active tuberculosis,[19,20] and nearly all pulmonologists were at some point patients in tuberculosis sanitaria.[21] Exposure to other incurable pathogens was also very common, and the public came to assume the existence of a professional "duty to treat." In modern surveys, 72% of Americans believe that it is a "doctor's obligation to treat all sick people".[22] All health care professionals, whether physicians, nurses, or paramedics, hold similar values with regard to the duty to treat, also called the "duty to care." This duty has become an integral part of what it means to be a health care professional.[23] Selfless service applies as well in other high-risk professions, such as public safety, law enforcement, and fire response.

Apart from professional integrity, several other ethical and practical bases for a duty to treat have been proposed, including professional virtue, patients' rights, social utility, and beneficence.[11,24–26] It has been argued, for example, that particular obligations arise from the special training medical professionals receive, which increases the value of their aid, reduces the risk associated with providing it, and might even reduce the chance that those without training will offer assistance.[26] If others are not available or cannot provide equally high-quality care, or if it would be riskier for others to try because they don't have the skills and training needed to protect themselves, then the moral obligation to step in and provide care is very strong. Because of this dynamic (referred to as *reliance*), acts of caring that might be considered heroic if done by a layperson should be seen as "all in a day's work" for health care professionals, who have been trained for, and are relied on, to perform. Finally, the U.S. Supreme Court has supported the duty to treat, in finding that discrimination against patients on the basis of an infectious disease can be a breach of the Americans With Disabilities Act in the case of Bragdon v Abbott, 524 US 624 (1998).

Despite these various reasons to live up to their responsibilities, actual experience, both historic and recent, has shown that some health care professionals flee in the face of danger.[27] During the SARS epidemic, medical staffing was difficult across nations due to work refusals by health care professionals.[5,28] This raises questions about the limits of the duty to treat and ways to buttress health care professionals' willingness to participate in disaster response.

5.6.1   Limits of Responsibilities

All patient care entails risk to the caregiver, often unrecognized. Still, risk-taking in patient care generally occurs across a spectrum. Care can be routine or heroic. At the far extreme, risk-taking is reckless. So the task is to set reasonable upper and lower limits on the duty to treat and other professional responsibilities. This recognizes the limits of human behavior.

When considering limits on the duty to treat, health care professionals have a competing obligation to ensure their own safety so that they can continue caring for other patients. This would preclude certain actions that might seem heroic, yet instead move closer to recklessness. Just as firefighters are trained to leave buildings before they collapse, health care professionals should not sacrifice themselves needlessly. However, the uncertain and fluctuating nature of medical risk can make such determinations very difficult or impossible.[12]

Between routine work and recklessness lies a great deal of space within which individuals must make decisions, taking into account competing duties (eg, to family) and individual characteristics (eg, special training and interest). Note that the more any duty is spelled out explicitly in advance and accepted by the specific actor, the greater the obligation to perform. Hence, not every health care professional holds the same duties.[29] Individuals choosing more risk-prone work or signing up for specific duties during crises have greater obligations.

Where health care professional services are greatly needed despite high risk, the duty to treat can be enforced through law. This occurred in China, Canada, and elsewhere during the SARS epidemic and is an option in the United States. State licensure statutes could be invoked to support continued care during emergencies. Federal law even allows US health care professionals to be drafted into national service in the event of a national catastrophe.[30] While a forcible draft of health care professionals would seem highly unlikely in our democratic society and could even prove counterproductive, the possibility highlights the legal recognition of the importance of continued health care professional service during crises.

Training health care professionals for disaster response should include discussions of the actual risks associated with typical scenarios. Health care professionals should also be trained in the use of personal protective equipment, as they have a responsibility to protect themselves.[25] It would be unfair for health care workers to reject a responsibility because it is too dangerous while refusing to take steps to lessen the danger.

By way of making expectations more explicit, the notion of offering danger pay, providing survivor benefits for the families of health care professionals who die or are injured in the line of duty, and naming special teams to address special risks are all valuable. It is also worthwhile for health care professionals taking on special risks to receive preferential access to reasonable countermeasures, such as vaccines and prophylactic therapies. This makes practical sense, because only healthy practitioners can help respond to any ongoing threat, and ethical sense, because reciprocity demands that those taking on extra risk on behalf of society receive special consideration from society to help mitigate the risk. Psychological support for caregivers is also important, since the toll of putting oneself and potentially one's family in danger can be harsh. After the SARS epidemic in Toronto, debilitating fears of infectious diseases were noted among some health care professionals, and enrollment in health professional schools declined.[5]

5.6.2   Reciprocity: Removing Barriers to Medical Volunteerism

Several important legal and practical barriers can impede medical volunteerism. For those injured during disaster response, the workers' compensation system is a patchwork that differs from state to state and even from one employer to another.[31] Most workers' compensation programs cover only employees, but some include volunteers. In some states, volunteers are defined as state employees during declared disasters. If temporarily defined as employees by an institution, volunteers may be eligible for benefits through that institution, but often a volunteer's existing employer is not liable for any injuries sustained in providing services outside the normal course of employment. One effort to address this issue is the Uniform Emergency Volunteer Health Professionals Act (UEVHPA), which was first promulgated by the National Conference of Commissioners on Uniform State Law in 2006. UEVHPA provisions are triggered by the declaration of an emergency by an authorized state or local official, remain in effect for the duration of that emergency, and apply to all licensed practitioners providing health or veterinary services. UEVHPA permits state governments to give reciprocity to volunteer practitioners licensed in other states, for provision during the emergency of services consistent with the disaster state's scope of practice for that practitioner, and without the volunteers otherwise meeting the disaster state's licensure requirements. In addition, under UEVHPA, volunteer health care practitioners who are injured or die as a result of providing services are deemed to be employees of the state for purposes of workers' compensation. Receiving compensation for services does not remove volunteers from protection by the Act, unless they are paid pursuant to a preexisting employment agreement. As of 2011, 11 states had adopted a version of the UEVHPA.[32]

In the United States, a barrier to volunteering across state lines has been the state-based professional licensure system. In declared disasters, licensure requirements can often be waived on the basis of an Emergency Management Assistance Compact. These were originally developed by the Southern Governors Association for southern states responding to hurricanes, but all 50 states now participate. The Compacts allow for sharing state-based resources in disasters, including personnel (medical and public health) and materiel. Also, federal health care providers licensed in one state can perform their official duties in any state. Federal providers include clinicians in the uniformed services, Veterans Affairs, and "federalized" workers serving on Disaster Medical Assistance Teams. A "federalized" worker has protection under the Federal Tort Claims Act from civil prosecution for adverse outcomes related to care provided under these circumstances. Under UEVHPA, volunteers who are registered, licensed, and in good standing in one state may practice in another state to the extent authorized, as if licensed in that state.

With regard to liability during disasters, regardless of the situation, there is no immunity from criminal liability (willful actions that cause harm). However, there can be immunity from civil liability, varying by state and according to mutual aid compacts, Good Samaritan statutes, and state emergency health powers statutes. Federalized providers (eg, those on Disaster Medical Assistance Teams) have civil immunity, but many other gaps remain for responders. The UEVHPA provides two alternative sections on immunity from civil liability for states to consider:

A: Complete immunity for volunteer practitioners and organizations under which they are utilized (host or deploying entity), regardless of volunteer compensation, for a volunteer practitioner's acts or omissions, unless the conduct is grossly negligent or criminal, or is the subject of a claim by the host or deploying entity; or

B: Complete immunity for volunteer practitioners, provided that volunteer compensation (for services provided in the emergency) is capped at $500 per year. Reasonable expenses are not included in this cap. Immunity under option "B" does not include the hosting organization (vicarious liability).

These options are best matched to existing state "Good Samaritan" liability protections and state implementation of relevant federal law.[33]

Finally, the responsibilities of health care professionals do not end with being willing to care for patients during public health emergencies.[10] There are also responsibilities to detect and report infectious diseases, for example, and to be trained in emergency response well enough that the health care professionals themselves do not contribute to the chaos of the situation. Spontaneous or freelance volunteerism by those untrained in the specific roles and responsibilities of disaster response can lead to a "mass provider incident," compounding resource shortages and exacerbating chaos.[34]

5.7 RESTRICTIONS

In 1907, an apparently healthy cook, Mary Mallon, was involuntarily admitted to the New York City Health Department's Detention Hospital. She was held there for three years as a carrier of typhoid fever. Prior to being released, she promised not to engage in any occupation that would bring her into contact with food, but she soon accepted a job as a cook at a hospital, causing dozens of cases of typhoid. She was again involuntarily committed, as public health officials concluded that only quarantine for the remainder of her life would effectively control the risk of typhoid transmission. "Typhoid Mary" died under quarantine.[35]

Although decisions about quarantine are generally made by those in the public health system, they are often implemented by clinicians and can affect the patient-clinician relationship.[9,36] Clinicians, therefore, should have a clear understanding of relevant public health laws and procedures, and the ethical basis underlying restrictions on individual liberties.

A range of individual rights can be curtailed during public health emergencies. For example, certain federal regulations may be waived when the president and the secretary of Health and Human Services declare a public health emergency. In particular, the Emergency Medical Treatment and Active Labor Act (EMTALA), which requires screening and stabilization of patients in emergency departments prior to transfer or discharge, can be waived for 72 hours. Several privacy rights mandated by the Health Insurance Portability and Accountability Act for patients within a health care facility may also be waived, including the requirement to obtain a patient's agreement to speak with family members or friends involved in the patient's care, to honor a request to opt out of the facility directory, to distribute a notice of privacy practices, to request privacy restrictions, and to request confidential communications.

While such restrictions on usual rights are important, the most extreme infringement on liberty for public health purposes is considered to be quarantine. *Quarantine* refers to the separation or restriction of movement of healthy persons who have been exposed, or who might have been exposed, to an infectious disease. *Isolation* is the separation of people who are already ill and presumed or known to be infected. Isolation is routinely used without much controversy for hospitalized patients with tuberculosis, chickenpox, bacterial meningitis, methicillin-resistant *Staphylococcus aureus* infection, influenza, and other infections, because the clinical rationale for isolation is often strong (eg, people with symptoms can be very contagious).

Since quarantine imposes sizeable costs on apparently healthy individuals and communities in terms of both liberty and economic effects, it requires strong ethical *and* clinical justifications. Ethically, it has been said that quarantine poses the starkest dilemma in all of public health ethics: pitting the ethos of civil liberties against that of public health. Remarkably, however, in some areas (notably, human immunodeficiency virus infection), a consensus to avoid quarantine has emerged because the public health community has agreed with civil libertarians that quarantine would probably be ineffective and could even drive infected patients away from care.[37]

In 1984 at Siracusa, Greece, the United Nations set out ethical principles that require consideration when enacting quarantine or any liberty-restricting measures. Actions should be "legitimate, legal, necessary, non-discriminatory and represent the least restrictive means appropriate to the reasonable achievement of public health goals."[38] Using the "least restrictive means" suggests that any limitations should be no more restrictive than necessary. Involuntary quarantine should not be used if voluntary "shelter-in-place" measures will work; restriction to one room should not be used if an entire house is available; visitors should be permitted if effective personal protective equipment is used; and if work can be continued from inside quarantine, then it should be permitted.[14] The idea is to preserve freedom and opportunity as far as possible, while still preventing significant risk of harm to others.

Others have stressed additional principles of reciprocity, proportionality, transparency, nondiscrimination, and accountability or due process.[7,13,39,40] All of these principles, however, are built on a single, primary ethical justification for quarantine, which is the general obligation not to harm others. As articulated by the original libertarian, John Stuart Mill in *On Liberty*, the "harm principle" is the notion that "the only purpose for which power can be rightfully exercised over any member of a civilized community, against his will, is to prevent harm to others."[41] Under this basic principle, quarantine could be just only if it prevents exposed people from infecting others.

This raises a central issue, however. Many people in quarantine will be exposed but not infected, which means they pose no danger to others. This is by far the most important dilemma related to quarantine. To be ethically acceptable, quarantine must first be effective at protecting the public's health. But is quarantine effective?

There is no simple answer to this question. The effectiveness of any particular quarantine action will depend on social characteristics (ie, whether the population accepts quarantine or rebels against it), biologic/disease characteristics (ie, transmissibility, duration of infectiousness, recovery rate, and symptom correlation with contagion), and individual characteristics (ie, whether individuals, both in and out of quarantine, adhere to infection control measures like wearing masks or avoiding public gatherings). However, the absence of a clear answer does not preclude strong opinions.

Some have asserted that the use of quarantine for SARS was "unnecessarily harmful" if not completely ineffective.[42] According to one account of the SARS epidemic in Taiwan, more than 131,000 people were placed under quarantine, and of these, only 12 became ill, and only two had confirmed cases of SARS.[5] Quoting Benjamin Franklin, George Annas has argued, "Those who would give up an essential liberty to purchase temporary security deserve neither liberty nor security."[5] He strongly warns against reorganizing public health on a military or police model (in which quarantine might be a part), as this would undermine public trust, promote fear and panic, and ultimately increase the spread of disease as frightened people break quarantine, flee, and disperse into the population.

To support these concerns, Annas notes that when a rumor spread that all of Beijing might be placed under quarantine for SARS, 245,000 migrant workers fled the city. Similarly, when Hong Kong's Amoy Gardens apartment complex (the site of an early SARS outbreak) was placed under quarantine, officials arriving to relocate residents found no one home in more than half of the complex's 264 apartments.[40] In fact, in every country that attempted to institute quarantine for SARS, violations occurred.[4] In Singapore, one individual was arrested when his picture showed up on the front page of the newspaper–a beer in one hand, his quarantine order in the other. As former Senator Sam Nunn (Democrat, Georgia) opined after participating in a tabletop exercise with a failed mass quarantine, "There is no force on earth that can make Americans do something that they do not believe is in their own best interests and that of their families".[40]

These examples show that quarantine done poorly can induce people to mistrust and avoid the public health system. A counter argument is that even if quarantine is not very effective, it might still be better than the alternatives. As a comparison, 14 million travelers were screened in China to find only 12 cases of SARS; more than 1 million people had their temperatures taken at Toronto airports without detecting a single SARS case. Worse yet, some clusters of cases in China were traced back to transmission that probably occurred while people were standing in line together, waiting to have their temperatures checked.[30] On the other hand, a recent study used mathematical models to demonstrate that even a very "leaky" quarantine could reduce the spread and duration of a pandemic flu epidemic.[43] Delaying infections can "smooth out" or widen the influenza epidemic curve, giving responders more time to prepare and alleviating strain on the system.[44] Finally, quarantine is sometimes considered when no effective treatments or vaccines are available, so its effectiveness is occasionally measured against a very short yardstick: doing nothing. That is the wrong way to look at it, however, since quarantine would not be used alone but in combination with other detection and containment strategies, such as social distancing methods, screening programs, and isolation of ill patients.

Equally important, the American public generally supports the use of quarantine. In a recent survey, 94% said they would comply with a 7- to 10-day voluntary quarantine if they were exposed in a pandemic flu.[45] This supports Paul Edelson's comment that "it is a canard sometimes used to justify authoritarian actions that the public responds to emergencies by losing control and panicking; indeed it is the consensus of social scientists that people in emergency situations tend to be more cooperative and more generous toward others than they may normally be."[35]

What the public worries about is that quarantine will be done poorly. Will those placed under quarantine be cared for well? Will they be recognized as making a sacrifice that is helping to protect the rest of the community, and for which they should receive respect, appreciation, and support? Will they receive food, salary replacement, and job security? Will they receive rapid medical care if they become ill, or prophylaxis if available? And if they are placed under quarantine outside the home, will someone care for their children, their pets, and their parents? In a recent four-nation survey about out-of-home quarantine, many people were concerned about overcrowding, cross-infection, and the inability to communicate with their families.[46] Almost 25% of Americans say they could not afford to miss work for a week, and nearly one in five say their employer would probably *require* them to work while ill, even if they might infect others.[44]

Researchers note that quarantine places a tremendous psychological strain on the quarantined individual and the community. In one study, symptoms of post-traumatic stress disorder and depression were seen in nearly one-third of those quarantined.[47] Others warn that quarantine has sometimes been used in discriminatory ways.[48,49] For example, a significant court ruling from 1900 noted that public health officials had acted with an "evil eye and an unequal hand" in placing an entire community of Chinese immigrants under quarantine in response to a plague scare.[39] Merely being in quarantine can lead to stigma, while confidentiality is almost impossible to maintain since the reasons for quarantine are generally well known.

Finally, while panic among the public is rare during public health crises, the same cannot be said with any certainty about political leaders. The urge to be perceived as responding aggressively might cause some to suggest the use of police- or military-enforced quarantines of broad populations, even when it might be useless or worsen the situation. Transparent communications, viewing the public as a partner, and attending to the ethical and practical issues that most concern the public are the best ways to ensure compliance with quarantine in a democracy.

5.8 RATIONING

When a Chiron plant was found to be producing contaminated flu vaccine in 2004, it was forced by British safety inspectors to close. With this move, the United States lost half its total vaccine supply for the 2004–2005 flu season, leading to dramatic shortfalls in many American clinics and hospitals. The federal government proposed a voluntary rationing scheme to distribute vaccines.[15]

What principles should drive resource allocation in disasters? The federal US plan for pandemic flu (available at http://www.hhs.gov/pandemicflu/plan/) endorses the prioritization guidance given by the National Vaccine Advisory Committee and the Advisory Committee on Immunization Practices. The specifics of the allocation guidance can change depending on the biological characteristics of the virus (transmissibility, mortality to different age groups), yet the general principle is to save the most lives possible given limited resources. Even this basic aim has received some ethical criticism. Alternative general principles might give very different priority to various groups (eg, children vs the elderly) if they operated on a principle of "save the most quality life-years" or "save those who are most needed" or "women and children first."

The most prominent critique of using a "save the most lives" principle comes from those advocating use of a "life-cycle allocation" (also called a "fair innings") principle.[50,51] This alternative would set a goal of ensuring that as many people as possible receive the opportunity to live through a full life cycle (ie, as many people as possible get to play the whole game of life, as in a nine-inning baseball game). According to Emanuel and Wertheimer, "there is great value in being able to pass through each life stage—to be a child, a young adult, and then to develop a career and family, and to grow old . . . ."[50] As a result, they recommend higher priority for people 13 to 40 years old who are otherwise healthy because they have more life stages yet to come. Incidentally, children received lowest priority for flu vaccination under earlier, hypothetical, federal pandemic flu vaccination guidance but high priority for actual H1N1 vaccination. This change was made because of unanticipated differences in risk of illness and death, however, not because of a change in the principle underlying the allocation strategy.

The fair innings approach to rationing has received its fair share of criticism, largely on the basis of its apparent ageism,[52,53] but it has intuitive appeal. In fact, prioritization of adults over children might spark a revolt among parents who would gladly give up their own vaccines so that their children could receive them. This practical dilemma raises an important issue about using any single general ethical principle to make allocation decisions.

The seeming advantage to having one basic goal to guide allocation decisions is that it can make tough decisions easier; once the goal is picked, whether most life stages or most lives, rationing is done by calculation. The problem is that real life is more complex than this. No actual allocation decisions or implementation plans are carried out by simple math. Instead, real-world allocation plans typically synthesize a number of different, sometimes conflicting, ethical principles and goals.[15]

For example, most prioritization plans place high priority on vaccine production and frontline health care workers. Many also seek to maintain public order by prioritizing key governmental and military personnel. Some explicitly aim at "minimizing societal and economic impacts."[54] These examples suggest that, like other areas where ethical "principlism" is used to guide policy decisions, it is rare for a single principle to trump all others.[55] Gostin proposed a set of eight criteria that all should be considered when rationing schemes are developed, to include protecting the most vulnerable, ensuring intergenerational equity, and promoting social justice.[56] One might also consider the importance of ensuring continuation of trust in society after the disaster, and providing comfort and respect for the dying.[15] Upshur and colleagues proposed 15 such principles across substantive and procedural values (Table 5-1).[8]

The main point is that, rather than acting as though a single ethical principle (eg, "save the most lives") is all one should consider in disasters, it is more helpful to recognize that multiple ethical principles must be considered. This more nuanced understanding also matches the reality of crisis planning and response, since providing care during disasters entails many complex decisions about how to do the best one can under severely constrained conditions.

TABLE 5-1 Principles for Public Health Crisis Planning

Substantive Value	Description
Individual liberty	In a public health crisis, restrictions to individual liberty should be proportional, necessary, and relevant; employ the least restrictive means; and be applied equitably.
Protection of the public from harm	In taking actions that impinge on individual liberty, decision makers should weigh the imperative for compliance; provide reasons for public health measures to encourage compliance; and establish mechanisms to review decisions.
Proportionality	Measures to protect the public from harm should not exceed what is necessary to address the actual level of risk to or critical needs of the community.
Privacy	In a public health crisis, it may be necessary to override the usual right to privacy in order to protect the public from serious harm.
Duty to provide care	Health care professionals have the duty to respond to suffering and to provide care, and may have to balance their professional demands with competing obligations to their own health and to family and friends.
Reciprocity	Society must support those who face a disproportionate burden in protecting the public good (health care workers, patients, and families) and take steps to reduce such burdens.
Equity	Under routine circumstances, all patients have an equal claim to receive the health care they need. During a health care crisis, the options available for care may vary from the routine: some services may be deferred.
Trust	Trust is an essential component of the relationships across clinicians and patients, within organizations, and between the public and health care providers, and among organizations within a health system. Maintaining trust while simultaneously implementing control measures during an evolving health care crisis is challenging.
Solidarity	A health care crisis calls for collaborative approaches that set aside traditional values of self-interest or territoriality among health care professionals, services, or institutions.
Stewardship	Decisions regarding resources are intended to achieve the best casualty and public health outcomes given the circumstances of the health crisis.
Procedural Value	Description
Reasonableness	Decisions should be evidence-based and grounded in values that are relevant to meeting health needs in a health crisis.
Openness and transparency	The decision-making process should be open to review and publicly accessible.
Inclusivity	Stakeholders should be able to engage in the decision-making process.
Responsiveness	The decision-making process should be able to adapt to emerging information, with mechanisms to address disputes.
Accountability	Decision makers should be answerable for their actions and inactions.

5.9 STANDARDS OF CARE IN DISASTERS

A productive way to plan for resource allocation in disasters is to consider how care delivery operations might need to change when resources (whether personnel, workspace, or material) are in short supply. This has sometimes been called the *altered standards of care* problem. This terminology can be misleading, however, since both legally and ethically, the "standard of care" always depends on the context of that care. In other words, the standard in medicine is to provide the best care reasonably attainable under the circumstances. Standards of care must be responsive to changing circumstances because it would be inappropriate to have a standard that is impossible to attain given the resources at hand. Recognizing this, state laws and ethical guidance are written to accommodate a standard of care based on the situation. Hence, there is not a single standard of care that will apply in every context.[57]

The context in a disaster is, by definition, very different from normal. Services reasonably expected under normal circumstances can be impossible to deliver during disasters. According to The Joint Commission, the aim in disasters is, when necessary, to ensure the "graceful degradation" in the quality of care provided. In September 2009, the Institute of Medicine (IOM) defined "crisis standards of care" as

> ... a substantial change in usual health care operations and the level of care it is possible to deliver, which is made necessary by a pervasive (e.g. pandemic influenza) or catastrophic (e.g. earthquake, hurricane) disaster. This change in the level of care delivered is justified by specific circumstances and is formally declared by a state government, in recognition that crisis operations will be in effect for a sustained period. The formal declaration that crisis standards of care are in operation enables specific legal/regulatory powers and protections for health care providers in the necessary tasks of allocating and using scarce medical resources and implementing alternate care site operations.

The IOM also provided a vision statement for providing care in disasters. One could argue that a similar vision should drive all health care resource allocation dilemmas, including noncrisis situations.[58,59] The IOM vision is to ensure that resource allocation decisions during disasters are recognized as fair by all those who might be affected. As such, the IOM did not lay out specific rules for resource allocation that should always apply nationwide, but instead emphasized the need to create equitable decision-making processes locally, which should be transparent, consistent, proportionate, and accountable. Local decision making facilitates participatory engagement by the community, which can help ensure the feasibility and acceptability of any rationing protocols, and allows for additional layers of accountability, authority, and legal due process.

This vision reflects a core set of ethical principles that can help guide allocation decisions. According to the IOM, these principles form a basic ethical framework that can be supplemented through local deliberations. There are three substantive norms—fairness, duty to care, and duty to steward shared resources—and four procedural norms—transparency, consistency, proportionality, and accountability.

Since the standard of care always depends on the context of that care, there is not one standard of care for all disasters. The challenge is to develop an ethical and legally supported process that enables disaster triage to achieve the goals of the community affected as fully as possible. Pre-event consideration of crisis standards of care within a community enlightens all within the community to this possibility. The IOM made six recommendations for developing crisis standards of care:

1. Develop consistent state crisis standards of care protocols with five key elements:
   ➤ Strong ethical grounds.
   ➤ Integrated and ongoing community and provider engagement, education, and communication.
   ➤ Assurances regarding legal authority and environment.
   ➤ Clear indicators, triggers, and lines of responsibility.
   ➤ Evidence-based clinical processes and operations.

2. Seek community and provider engagement

3. Adhere to ethical norms during crisis standards of care

4. Provide necessary legal protection for health care practitioners and institutions implementing crisis standards of care

5. Ensure consistency in crisis standards of care implementation

6. Ensure intrastate and interstate consistency among neighboring jurisdictions

Additional values or principles that might be considered by communities include a formal process/analysis to confirm that rationing is necessary; specific efforts to protect the vulnerable in society (eg, homeless, mentally ill, poor, language minorities); promotion of social justice, such as ensuring equal access to transportation away from the area; maintenance of social order, such as by prioritizing police and firefighters for early care or preventive measures; minimizing economic impact, such as prioritizing certain classes of workers like mail/delivery people and computer technologists (to facilitate telecommuting); ensuring continuation of a good society, such as treating people as we would wish to be treated, fostering respect, and paying attention to the reality that people will need to live together after the disaster passes; and respect for the dying, such as not placing those expected to die with those already dead, and providing adequate pain relief to those triaged to expectant care.

The dilemma of triage for expectant care (comfort care only) deserves special attention. Triage to expectant care involves two groups: those with absolutely unsalvageable injuries even under the best of circumstances and those with relatively unsalvageable injuries in the setting of scarce resources. The ethical basis for providing only comfort care to those with severe injuries during resource shortages rests on the necessity of doing so to ensure that others will live. In its starkest terms, the problem is that two casualties can require a certain resource for survival, whether staff time, a ventilator, a drug, or anything else in short supply. When this is true, the decision maker—often a health care professional—faces a classic "Sophie's choice" (a forced choice between two unbearable options): no matter who receives the resource, the other will die. In this situation, if one casualty is more likely to die even with access to the scarce resource, that factor can tilt the ethical balance.

Recognizing intellectually that this is a forced choice and a no-win situation with no good options does not prevent deep discomfort with facing it. Yet health care professionals should recognize that withdrawal of care, palliative care, and expectant care provided under these circumstances are not the same as euthanasia. First, euthanasia is intentional killing, not withdrawal of care. Second, euthanasia implies that a meaningful choice not to participate in a death exists, but in this situation all choices lead to someone's death. When circumstances do not allow for all patients to receive all the care that could provide substantial benefit, it is not unethical to withhold or withdraw resources from those least likely to benefit so that others might survive. In fact, many might argue that it would be unethical not to do so.

The entire ethical argument for allowing expectant care during disasters hinges, however, on some critical caveats. Most importantly, the person making these decisions must have excellent "situational awareness," including awareness of what resources are available, when, and where. An ad hoc decision maker could easily believe a casualty is unsalvageable given available resources, without being aware that additional resources are available nearby or are to become available soon. Such decisions also demand wisdom, care, and thoughtfulness—these are not decisions that should be made on the fly by clinicians operating on 48 hours without sleep. Similarly, as situations change, a previously determined unsalvageable casualty might improve, or new resources might alter the determination, or a casualty previously thought to have good odds might do worse than expected. It is critical that allocation decisions be formally revisited on a regular basis as the crisis evolves. Also, the intent of comfort care is just that: comfort. Those triaged to expectant care deserve dignity and respect.

Finally, significant concerns remain about criminalizing decisions about expectant care when medical personnel and supplies are severely compromised. The AMA and the American Nurses Association have emphasized jointly that during any disaster, health care providers—physicians, nurses, and others—must be able to work together to make the best decisions given available resources;[59] post hoc criminal prosecution fosters fear of having best judgments second-guessed in disasters and could hinder an effective response.

5.10 SUMMARY

Legal structures for disaster response affirm that effective disaster response is first local, then moves in stages to state and federal resources. Ethically, considering three R's (responsibilities, restrictions, and rationing) can help to focus thinking on dominant ethical issues in disaster planning and response. Responsibilities of health care professionals around disaster response include the duty to care for those affected and reciprocal obligations of society to protect those serving in disasters; support for restrictions on individual liberties, such as isolation and quarantine, when necessary to protect the larger community while assuring respect for affected individuals; and rationing decisions made through crisis care operations that are different from normal operations, yet that are based on the same ethical principles that govern usual care.[60]

REFERENCES

1. Subbarao I, Lyznicki J, Hsu E, et.al., A consensus-based educational framework and competency set for the discipline of disaster medicine and public health preparedness. *Disaster Med Public Health Prep.* 2008;2:57–68.

2. Camus A. *The Plague.* New York, NY: Vintage Books; 1991.

3. Emanuel EJ. The lessons of SARS. *Ann Intern Med.* 2003;139:589–591.

4. Branswell H. SARS continues to exact mental toll on shell-shocked health-care workers. *The Guardian.* December 31, 2003: E9.

5. Rothstein MA, Alcalde MG, Elster NR, et al. *Quarantine and Isolation: Lessons Learned From SARS: A Report to the Centers for Disease Control and Prevention.* Louisville, KY: Institute for Bioethics, Health Policy, and Law, University of Louisville School of Medicine; November 2003:20. http://www.louisville.edu/medschool/ibhpl/publications/SARS%20REPORT.pdf

6. Garrett L; Council on Foreign Relations. Avian flu update. http://www.cfr.org/publication/9018/avian_flu_update.html. Accessed November 22, 2009.

7. Shaffer D, Armstrong G, Higgins K, et al. Increased US prescription trends associated with the CDC *Bacillus anthracis* antimicrobial postexposure prophylaxis campaign. *Pharmacoepidemiol Drug Saf.* 2003;12:177–182.

8. Upshur R, Faith K, Gibson JL, et al. *Stand on Guard for Thee: Ethical Considerations in Preparedness Planning for Pandemic Influenza.* Toronto, Ontario, Canada: University of Toronto Joint Center for Bioethics; 2005. http://www.jointcentreforbioethics.ca/people/documents/upshur_stand_guard.pdf. Accessed November 22, 2009.

9. Berlinger N, Moses J. The five people you meet in a pandemic—and what they need from you today. *Hastings Center Bioethics Backgrounder* [serial online]. 2007. http://www.thehastingscenter.org/uploadedFiles/Publications/Special_Reports/Pandemic-Backgrounder-The-Hastings-Center.pdf. Accessed November 22, 2009.

10. Wynia MK, Gostin LO. Ethical challenges in preparing for bioterrorism: barriers within the health care system. *Am J Public Health.* 2004;94:1096–1102.

11. Huber SJ, Wynia MK. When pestilence prevails: physician responsibilities in epidemics. *Am J Bioethics*. 2004;4:5–11.

12. Wynia MK. Ethics and public health emergencies: encouraging responsibility. *Am J Bioethics*. 2007; 7:1–4.

13. Brody H, Avery EN. Medicine's duty to treat pandemic illness: solidarity and vulnerability. *Hastings Center Rep*. 2009;39:40–48.

14. Wynia MK. Ethics and public health emergencies: restrictions on liberty. *Am J Bioethics*. 2007;7:1–5.

15. Wynia MK. Ethics and public health emergencies: rationing vaccines. *Am J Bioethics*. 2006;6:4–7.

16. Fink S. Strained by Katrina, a hospital faced deadly choices. *New York Times Magazine*. August 30, 2009. http://www.nytimes.com/2009/08/30/magazine/30doctors.html. Accessed November 22, 2009.

17. Jonsen A. *A Short History of Medical Ethics*. New York, NY: Oxford University Press; 2000.

18. Bell J, Hayes I. Code of ethics. In: Baker RB, Caplan AL, Emanuel LL, Latham SR, eds. *The American Medical Ethics Revolution*. Appendix C. Baltimore, MD: Johns Hopkins University Press; 1999.

19. Myers J. The natural history of tuberculosis in the human body. *JAMA*. 1965;194:1086–1092.

20. Sepkowitz K. Occupationally acquired infections in health care workers: part II. *Ann Intern Med*. 1996;125:917–928.

21. Snider G. Tuberculosis then and now: a personal perspective on the last 50 years. *Ann Intern Med*. 1997;126: 237–243.

22. Roper Center for Public Opinion Research. *Great American TV Poll #4*. Princeton, NJ: Princeton Survey Research Associates; 1991.

23. Altevogt B, Stroud C, Hanson SL, et al. *Guidance for Establishing Crisis Standards of Care for Use in Disaster Situations* [book online]. Washington, DC: Institute of Medicine, National Academies Press; 2009. http://books.nap.edu/openbook.php?record_id=12749&page=R2. Accessed November 22, 2009.

24. White CC. Health care professionals and treatment of HIV-positive patients: is there an affirmative duty to treat under common law, the Rehabilitation Act, or the Americans with Disabilities Act? *J Leg Med*. 1999;20:67–113.

25. American Medical Association Council on Ethical and Judicial Affairs. Physician obligation in disaster preparedness and response—recommendations. 2004. http://www.ama-assn.org/ama1/pub/upload/mm/code-medical-ethics/9067a.pdf. Accessed January 9, 2007.

26. Clark CC. Of epidemic proportions: physicians, public trust and personal risk. *Yale J Biol Med*. 2005;78:363–372.

27. Zuger A, Miles SH. Physicians, AIDS, and occupational risk: historic traditions and ethical obligations. *JAMA*. 1987;258:1924–1928.

28. Altman L. Asian medics stay home, imperiling respirator patients. *New York Times*. March 21, 2003: A6.

29. Iserson KV, Heine CE, Larkin GL, Moskop JC, Baruch J, Aswegan AL. Fight or flight: the ethics of emergency physician disaster response. *Ann Emerg Med*. April 2008;51:345–353.

30. Pear R. US has contingency plans for a draft of medical workers. *New York Times*. October 19, 2004. http://www.nytimes.com/2004/10/19/politics/19draft.html?ex=1255924800&en=0dac35afc2209e66&ei=5088&partner=rssnyt. Accessed January 12, 2007.

31. Hoffman S, Goodman R, Stier D. Law, liability, and public health emergencies. *Disaster Med Public Health Prep*. 2009;3:117–125.

32. Walters A, The UEVHPA: An Update. Bulletin of the American College of Surgeons, May 2010, pp. 28–29.

33. http://www.uevhpa.org, accessed on April 15, 2011.

34. Larkin GLL. Unwitting partners in death: The ethics of teamwork in disaster response. *Virtual Mentor*. 2010;12:495–501. http://virtualmentor.ama-assn.org/2010/06/oped1-1006.html. Accessed July 12, 2010.

35. Edelson PJ. Quarantine and civil liberties. In: Balint J, Philpott S, Baker R, Strosberg M, eds. *Ethics and Epidemics*. Amsterdam, the Netherlands: Elsevier Press; 2006.

36. Annas GJ. Bioterrorism, public health, and civil liberties. *N Engl J Med*. 2002;346:1337–1342.

37. Bayer R, Fairchild-Carrino A. AIDS and the limits of control: public health orders, quarantine, and recalcitrant behavior. *Am J Public Health*. 1993;83:1471–1476.

38. United Nations Economic and Social Council, UN Sub-Commission on Prevention of Discrimination and Protection of Minorities. Siracusa Principles on the Limitation and Derogation of Provisions in the International Covenant on Civil and Political Rights UN Doc E/CN.4/1984/4 (Annex). http://hei.unige.ch/~clapham/hrdoc/docs/siracusa.html. Accessed November 3, 2006.

39. American Medical Association Council on Ethical and Judicial Affairs. The use of quarantine and isolation as public health interventions. *CEJA Opin*. 2006;1-A-06.

40. Gostin LO, Bayer R, Fairchild AL. Ethical and legal challenges posed by severe acute respiratory syndrome. *JAMA*. 2003;290:3229–3237.

41. Mill JS. *On Liberty* [book online]. 1859. http://www.utilitarianism.com/ol/one.html. Accessed November 3, 2006.

42. Annas GJ. Bioterror and "bioart"—a plague o' both your houses. *N Engl J Med*. 2006;354:2715–2720.

43. Wu JT, S Riley, C Fraser, GM Leung. Reducing the impact of the next influenza pandemic using household-based public health interventions. *PloS Med*. 2006;3:e361. dx.doi.org/10.1371/journal.pmed.0030361. Accessed October 31, 2006.

44. Doney M. Nonpharmaceutical public health interventions: strategies and implementation in the setting of pandemic influenza. In: Presentation August 26, 2006. http://www.bt.cdc.gov/coca/ppt/COCA_NPPHI_borders_communities_Pan_Flu.ppt. Accessed November 3, 2006.

45. Blendon RJ, Benson JM, Weldon KJ, Herrmann MJ. Pandemic influenza and the public: survey findings. Presented to the Institute of Medicine; October 26, 2006. http://www.hsph.harvard.edu/press/releases/press10262006.html. Accessed November 1, 2006.

46. Blendon RJ, DesRoches CM, Cetron MS, Benson JM, Meinhardt T, Pollard W. Attitudes toward the use of quarantine in a public health emergency in four countries. *Health Affairs*. 2006;25:w15–w25.

47. Hawryluck L, Gold WL, Robinson S, Pogorski S, Galea S, Styra R. SARA control and psychological effects of quarantine, Toronto, Canada. *Emerging Infect Dis*. 2004;10:1206–1212.

48. Reis N. The 2003 SARS outbreak in Canada: legal and ethical lessons about the use of quarantine. In: Balint J, Philpott S, Baker R, and Strosberg M, eds. *Ethics and Epidemics*. Amsterdam, the Netherlands: Elsevier Press; 2006.

49. Parmet WE. AIDS and quarantine: the revival of an archaic doctrine. *Hofstra Law Rev*. 1985–1986;53.

50. Emanuel EJ, Wertheimer A. Who should get influenza vaccine when not all can? *Science*. 2006;312:854–855.

51. Stolk EA, Pickee SJ, Ament AH, Buschbach JJ. Equity in health care prioritization: an empirical inquiry into social value. *Health Policy*. November 2005;74:343–355.

52. Rivlin MM. Why the fair innings argument is not persuasive. *BMC Med Ethics* [serial online]. 2000;1:E1.

53. Nord E. Concerns for the worse off: fair innings versus severity. *Soc Sci Med.* January 2005;60:257–263.

54. National Vaccine Advisory Committee, Advisory Committee on Immunization Practices. July 19, 2005:D19.

55. Wynia MK. Public health principlism: the precautionary principle and beyond. *Am J Bioethics.* 2005;5:3–4.

56. Gostin LO. Medical countermeasures for pandemic influenza; ethics and the law. *JAMA.* 2006;295:554–556.

57. Annas GJ. Standard of care—in sickness and in health and in emergencies. *N Engl J Med.* 2010;362:2126–2131.

58. Daniels N, Sabin JE. Making insurance coverage for new technologies reasonable and accountable. *JAMA.* 1998;279:703–704.

59. Wynia MK, Cummins D, Fleming D, et al, writing for the Oversight Body of the Ethical Force Program. Improving fairness in coverage decisions: performance expectations for quality improvement. *Am J Bioethics.* 2004;4(3):87–100.

60. Bristol N. Practitioner liability protections approved. *Disaster Med Public Health Prep.* 2007;1:73–75.

CHAPTER | SIX

Personal Protective Equipment and Casualty Decontamination

Greene Shepherd, PharmD

Richard B. Schwartz, MD

6.1 PURPOSE

This chapter reviews decontamination techniques and types of personal protective equipment (PPE) that may be required during a disaster with biologic, chemical, and radiologic hazards. Most health care workers already are familiar with basic PPE known as *universal precautions*. However, health care workers involved with a disaster are often challenged by threats and hazards that are different from those encountered during a normal workday and thus require additional or different PPE.[1-4] The exact type of equipment that will be available for use during an event will vary from place to place based on local resources, hazard assessment and preplanning.

6.2 LEARNING OBJECTIVES

➤ Describe wet, dry, and contaminant-specific decontamination techniques.

➤ Discuss the requirements for decontamination of ambulatory casualties.

➤ Differentiate levels of personal protection based on exposure risk.

➤ Demonstrate proper donning and doffing procedures for level C protection.

6.3   DISASTER MEDICINE AND PUBLIC HEALTH PREPAREDNESS COMPETENCIES ADDRESSED[5]

➤ Use federal and institution guidelines and protocols to prevent the transmission of infectious agents in health care and community settings. (4.1.4)

➤ Demonstrate the ability to select, locate, don, and work in PPE according to the degree and type of protection required for various types of exposures. (4.2.2)

➤ Explain the purpose of casualty decontamination in a disaster. (4.3.1)

6.4   CONTAMINATION

Contamination of casualties and health care providers with hazardous materials can occur in the course of daily health care or as a result of natural or manmade disasters. Hazardous materials can cause a wide variety of injuries ranging from mild irritation to life-threatening emergencies. The specific hazard presented by a contaminant depends on how it may affect the body, the physical state of the substance, the amount present, and the mode of release.

Physical Characteristics of Contaminants

➤ Aerosols, vapors, and gases affect casualties more rapidly than liquids or solids. They are, however, generally easier to remove from the casualty and will often dissipate before casualty movement.[6]

➤ Liquids tend to act on the site where they contact the skin and are harder to remove. A highly liquid-contaminated casualty poses more risk to responders/receivers than one with minimal contamination, and will be more difficult to decontaminate.

➤ Solid chemicals are much less reactive and are of low risk as a dermal hazard, but respirable particles are a respiratory hazard. Powders should be brushed off before the casualties are washed because wetting them enables chemical reactions. The smaller the particle size, the more difficult it will be to decontaminate.

In gas or liquid form many chemicals can cause irritation or burns on contact, while others may affect the body like a drug and alter physiologic processes (heart rate, blood pressure, or fluid secretion). Solid particulates (such as silica or asbestos) smaller than 10 μm can produce acute or chronic respiratory ailments. Contamination with radioactive chemicals in any state of matter presents a unique hazard that may not be readily apparent. Infectious materials can be spread by a variety of methods. Several classes of pathogens can cause infection, including bacteria, viruses, fungi, parasites, and prions. The modes of transmission vary by type of organism, with some infectious agents being transmitted by more than one route: some are transmitted primarily by direct or indirect contact (eg, herpes simplex virus, respiratory syncytial virus, *Staphylococcus aureus*) and others by the droplet (eg, influenza virus, *Bordetella pertussis*) or airborne (eg, *Mycobacterium tuberculosis*) route. Importantly, not all infectious agents are readily transmitted from person to person. Other infectious agents, such as blood-borne viruses (eg, hepatitis B and C viruses and human immunodeficiency virus), are transmitted rarely in health care settings, via percutaneous or mucous membrane exposure.

In addition to the direct hazard a substance poses to a casualty, there is a risk of secondary contamination of other people. Preventing hazard transmission from contaminated casualties to workers and other casualties (secondary contamination) is one of the most important features of medical response to chemical, radiologic, and biologic threats. Figures 6-1 and 6-2 list the methods of transmission of chemical and biologic hazards.

Spread of contamination can be minimized by the following actions:

➤ *Avoidance:* limit direct contact with contaminant if possible.

➤ *Protective equipment:* wear barrier garments to prevent self-contamination.

➤ *Good technique:* limit transfer and spread of contaminant on PPE.

➤ *Decontamination*

    ➣ Removal: remove contaminated clothing.

    ➣ Dilution: reduce concentration of harmful substances to safe levels with water.

FIGURE 6-1
Methods of Chemical
Hazard Transmission

Method	Example
• Transfer: move from one surface to another	→ Casualty to worker
• Spread: spread of contamination on same surface	→ Contaminated hand touches clean face
• Desorption: absorbed liquid gives off vapor	→ Chemical agent trapped in porous material off-gases
• Vapor and aerosol: carried through air	→ Casualty off-gassing

FIGURE 6-2
Methods of Biologic
Hazard Transmission

Method	Example
• Direct contact: casualty body fluids to worker	→ Enters via mucous membranes or broken skin
• Indirect contact: contaminated intermediate	→ Hand or object spreads to another person
• Respiratory droplet: cough, sneeze, or talking	→ Contact hazard expelled up to 6 feet
• Airborne: droplet or particle	→ Carried through the air over long distances

> ➤ Absorption: pick up spilled substances with an inert absorbent material.

> ➤ Degradation: alter chemical structure of harmful substance with an active chemical agent.

➤ *Isolation:* bag and clearly identify materials that cannot be successfully decontaminated. Casualties with infectious diseases that are easily transmitted should be isolated in rooms with appropriate environmental controls.

➤ *Disposal:* Move harmful substances to an approved disposal site.

When methods for preventing secondary contamination are selected, considerations include the type and amount of contaminant present, as well as the available resources and type of protective equipment needed to safely perform the task.

6.5   DECONTAMINATION

In a mass casualty decontamination event, it is estimated that only 20% of people will have clinically significant contamination.[2] However, all who present as casualties will require evaluation and some form of decontamination. The majority of casualties will self-refer to hospitals and arrive without formal decontamination. Initially, ambulatory casualties will self-transport. Later in the event, non-ambulatory casualties will arrive, are more likely to have been transported by emergency medical services (EMS). However, it should not be assumed that they have been decontaminated just because they were transported by EMS.

For small events, such as a single worker who is contaminated with a chemical spill, decontamination is typically performed by emergency department personnel who have had decontamination training. Mass casualty decontamination is logistically more demanding and is a process that requires trained decontamination teams that are made up of both clinical and nonclinical trained personnel. For mass casualty events where decontamination is required, it is prudent to conserve clinical personnel by staffing a majority of decontamination positions with nonclinical personnel. Clinical personnel should remain engaged for triage and emergent treatment. Relying solely on clinical staff to perform mass casualty decontamination diminishes resources for post-decontamination care and non-contaminated casualties. Just-in-time formation of decontamination teams puts personnel at risk: decontamination team members should be identified prior to an event and should receive education and training. Practice through team drills is essential for demonstrating the ability to perform mass casualty decontamination and should involve a realistic number of casualties. Decontamination at the hospital must not be outsourced to public safety organizations, such as the fire department: these organizations will be otherwise occupied in the setting of a disaster.

Decontamination of casualties who present to health care facilities consists of two basic methods.[1] The first, involving disrobing of potentially or grossly contaminated casualties, is commonly called *dry decontamination*. The same term, *dry decontamination*, is also occasionally used to describe the use of a dry powder or resin to remove contaminants. In NDLS, the term is used to mean simply the act of removing garments that are superficially contaminated or have retained vapor within them. The second method washes the grossly contaminated and/or symptomatic casualty from head to toe with detergent and tepid water and is called *wet decontamination*.

Although dry decontamination may seem like a simple thing, it is a major intervention that reduces possible hazard transmission. During the medical response to the 1995 Tokyo subway sarin attack, 23% of health workers were affected by contamination. However, once disrobing of ambulatory patients outside of the facility was initiated, there was no further contamination of health care workers.[7] It is estimated that if the casualty is fully clothed when exposed to contaminant, disrobing will remove the majority of contamination.[1,2,6] Dry decontamination is appropriate for casualties who have been exposed to gases or aerosol/vapors and have no more than minor respiratory effects.[1] However, casualties with significant skin or mucus membrane irritation or burns should undergo wet decontamination, even if the hazard is thought to be a vapor. It is possible to dry decontaminate large numbers of casualties very quickly; however, this does require planning and can be difficult from a logistical perspective. Ideally, it would occur in a large area with methods in place to provide crowd control, privacy (with separation of males and females during undressing and dressing), isolation of contaminated garments, and clean clothes.

The process of wet decontamination consists of disrobing the casualty and showering/washing under low pressure with tepid water and a sponge or washcloth.[1] Brushes with stiff bristles should be avoided because of the potential for skin abrasion. Mild detergent should be used to decontaminate the casualty. Military units will sometimes use a dilute bleach solution for casualty decontamination; however, this is not recommended for the civilian setting where large volumes of water are available and the addition of bleach or other harsh chemicals may actually potentiate tissue injury. Using tepid water is important because water that is too hot promotes toxin absorption, and water that is too cold is less effective at the removal of contaminants and may lead to hypothermia. Casualties should wash in a systematic manner from head to toe, starting first around the mouth and nose and around open wounds and lasting ideally for 3 to 5 minutes. Casualties who are unconscious or otherwise unable to wash themselves should be washed by a team of two to four people in appropriate protective equipment and in the same systematic manner. When overhead showers are used, water may enter an unconscious patient's airway; the face, head, and neck may need to be decontaminated first and the airway protected from water during the decontamination process. Careful attention should be paid to washing the recesses and creases, such as the ears, eyes, axillae, and groin, and to rolling the casualty over for washing the back. Performing wet decontamination has logistical challenges even greater than those described for dry decontamination: it requires additional resources (eg, water, power, runoff containment) and more personnel.

Decontamination can be performed near the area of release by fire or HAZMAT teams using low-pressure water from fire hoses or portable decontamination shelters.[2] However, due to the time delay necessary for setting up on-scene decontamination sites, most patients will likely present to hospitals for decontamination rather than waiting at the scene to be decontaminated. Ideally, the location for performing mass casualty decontamination at a hospital would be far enough away from normal treatment areas to prevent contamination of other patients, workers, and the facility itself. The site should be downwind and downhill from the health care facility. Obviously, these ideal requirements are not always logistically possible, and the location of the site must balance the principles of decontamination with the characteristics of the physical plant. The mass casualty decontamination area will require approximately 0.5 to 1 acre. It should include clearly delineated contaminated and clean areas. Triage, immediate treatments, and casualty and technical (personnel) decontamination will occur in the contaminated areas. Clean areas will be used for staging, worker rehabilitation, and casualty transfer/registration. A sample site layout can be seen in Figure 6-3. Approximately 20 people will be required to staff a mass casualty decontamination area. Approximately 10 to 12 people dressed in PPE will be needed for the contaminated area and another 10 people (capable of wearing PPE if needed) will be needed in support roles for the clean area.

The ingress and egress routes should also be controlled and coordinated with public safety agencies. The decontamination site should not impede normal

FIGURE 6-3
Mass Casualty
Decontamination Area

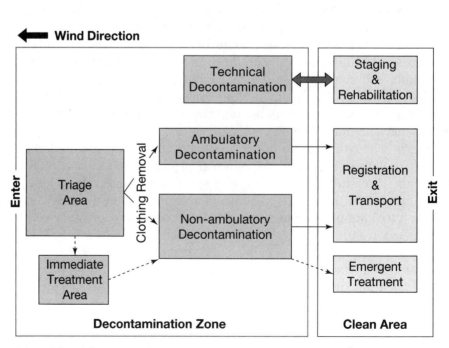

Adapted from US Army and Soldier and Biological Chemical Command.[2]

ambulance traffic. The area will need access to utilities (lights, water, and power) and should provide shelter. The ground surface should be reasonably flat and paved, if possible, to prevent contamination into the ground. Runoff should be controlled, and there must be a plan for managing contaminated waste water.

In cold environments, wet decontamination presents additional challenges in terms of patient safety and logistical requirements. Regardless of the ambient temperature, people who have been exposed to a known life-threatening level of chemical contamination should undergo decontamination and be sheltered as soon as possible.[8] If the external temperature is less than 65 °F (18 °C), casualties become at risk for hypothermia during or after the wet decontamination process. Wind chill must also be taken into account, as body heat is lost at a greater rate as wind speed increases. Cold water causes heat loss 26 times faster than ambient air of the same temperature.[8] Therefore, heated water must be used in cold environments. Figure 6-4 describes changes to normal decontamination procedures based on decreasing temperatures. In cold weather, casualties should be monitored for signs and symptoms of hypothermia before, during, and after the decontamination process. At body temperatures lower than 98 °F (37 °C), people will feel cold and shiver; at less than 95 °F (35 °C) physical and mental impairment begin; and at 86 °F (30 °C) shivering stops and loss of consciousness occurs.

Decontamination operations are complex, resource-intense endeavors that should not be underestimated. It is a process that requires planning and must account for real human behavior and difficult logistical considerations (Table 6-1).

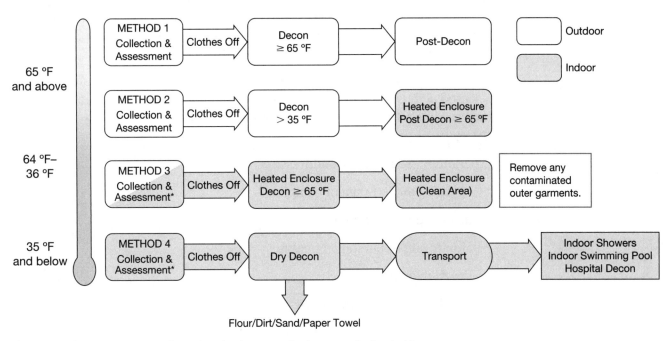

Collection refers to weapons, equipment, and outer garments. *Assessment* refers to triage.

FIGURE 6-4 Selection of Appropriate Patient Decontamination During Cold Weather[8]

TABLE 6-1 10 Considerations for Proposed Decontamination Sites

Is there enough space at the proposed site?
Where are the decontamination logistics located relative to the proposed site?
Are there appropriate traffic routes adjacent to the proposed site?
Is the proposed site in proximity to the point of casualty entry into the hospital without compromising care of non-contaminated/decontaminated casualties?
What is the water source for the proposed site?
What is the drainage from the proposed site?
How are contaminated clothes managed from the site?
How are potentially contaminated casualties triaged before and after decontamination?
How is security maintained at the site?
What is the impact of weather (eg, wind, rain, ambient light) at the site?

6.6 PERSONAL PROTECTIVE EQUIPMENT (PPE)

The importance of protective equipment for worker safety is widely recognized, and such equipment is required under federal laws and regulations promulgated by the US Occupational Safety and Health Administration (OSHA). OSHA has established regulations for workers involved in hazardous waste operations and emergency response. These regulations can be found in the *Code of Federal Regulations* in 29 CFR 1910-120 and 29 CFR 1910-134.[9,10]

➤ 29 CFR 1910-120 requires that appropriate protective equipment shall be selected and used to protect employees from hazards and potential hazards they are likely to encounter on the basis of a risk assessment.

➤ CFR 1910.134 describes OSHA's requirements for a respiratory protection program. A program must address:

➢ Cleaning and storage of equipment.

➢ Inspection of equipment.

➢ Monitoring of personnel health.

➢ Program evaluation.

➢ Physical fitness of employees.

➢ Respirators that are appropriate for the duty.

➢ Medical monitoring and evaluation.

Prior to fit-testing or respirator use, employers are required to provide a medical evaluation for workers who will use a respirator in the workplace. Screening forms may be used for operations-level workers and followed up with pulmonary function tests or a physical examination as the physician deems necessary. For HAZMAT team members and hazardous material specialists, examination by a physician is required. The employer may discontinue an employee's medical evaluations when the employee is no longer required to use a respirator.

The OSHA Respiratory Protection Standards, in 29 CFR 1910.134(e) or the parallel State Plan standards, require employers to obtain, in writing, a medical opinion regarding an employee's ability to wear a respirator. This evaluation should occur at least annually. An additional medical evaluation is required by paragraph 1910.134(e)(7), under certain circumstances. Prior to an incident, hospitals should conduct a thorough baseline evaluation of an employee's health to include allergies and current medications at the time the person is hired and any follow-up evaluations needed. Evaluations for medical clearance to wear a respirator should be incorporated into these examinations. A history of asthma or claustrophobia may preclude safe and effective use of PPE. On the basis of local policy, the employee's job category, or the hazards associated with tasks the employee performs, additional periodic health monitoring might also be provided. If necessary, it is possible to use personnel without a formal medical evaluation when participation has not been previously anticipated, provided that they are given a briefing at the site that includes instruction on PPE use, chemical hazards and assigned duties, and site safety precautions provided for the rest of the team.[10] Immediately before and after dressing out, each worker should undergo monitoring of weight and vital signs (pulse, blood pressure, temperature, and respirations) to assess heat stress and overall health as described in Section 6.6.2.[1,9] Additional follow-up is necessary for workers who sustain any exposure or other health problem during the operational period.

These regulations provide the framework for safe application of PPE and emphasize that use of PPE requires forethought and systems-thinking.

6.6.1   Heat Stress and PPE

Higher levels of PPE (above level D— see below) limit the body's ability to cool down; consequently, one of the greatest risks to health care workers using PPE during a disaster response is heat stress. Heat stress can range from heat rash and cramps to heat exhaustion and stroke. In addition to the type of PPE being worn, age, weight, degree of physical fitness, degree of acclimatization, metabolism, use of alcohol or drugs, and a variety of medical conditions can affect a person's sensitivity to heat.[11,12] A history of heat injury predisposes an individual to additional injury. It is difficult to predict who will be affected and when, because individual susceptibility varies. In addition, there is an interplay with environmental factors beyond ambient air temperature. Radiant heat, air movement, conduction, and relative humidity all affect an individual's response to heat. Research indicates that each 1% of the body's fluid that is lost will raise the core temperature by about 0.14 to 0.28 °C.[11] A 5% loss of fluid volume will impair the ability to sweat (and thus cool oneself) and decrease performance by as much as 50%.[11]

Heat stroke is a medical emergency and occurs when the body's system of temperature regulation fails and body temperature rises to critical levels. This condition is caused by a combination of highly variable factors, and its occurrence is difficult to predict. The primary signs and symptoms of heat stroke are progressive confusion, irrational behavior, loss of consciousness, and convulsions; a lack of sweating (usually) and hot, dry skin; and an abnormally high body temperature, eg, a rectal temperature of 105.8 °F (41 °C). When heat stroke is suspected, prompt medical attention is required. The heat casualty should be rapidly moved to a shaded area, disrobed, and cooled. Cooling can be achieved by wetting and fanning to promote evaporative cooling, application of ice packs or cooling vests, or administration of cool oral or intravenous fluids.

Heat exhaustion presents as fatigue, headache, nausea, vertigo, weakness, thirst, giddiness, and fainting. Fainting episodes may be due to increased body temperature or pooling of blood in extremities as the body attempts to cool off. The effects associated with heat exhaustion can be dangerous to others if the heat casualty is operating machinery. Acclimatization and active fluid replacement will help prevent these effects from occurring. When heat exhaustion occurs, it responds readily to prompt treatment. Workers sustaining heat exhaustion should be moved to a shaded area and given fluid replacement. They should also be encouraged to get adequate rest.

Heat cramps occur when working in a hot environment and represent an electrolyte imbalance caused by sweating: too much or too little salt. Most commonly, cramps appear to be caused by poor rehydration in the setting of sweat (sweat is hypotonic at 0.3% sodium chloride), leading to elevated serum concentrations of sodium and chloride. Thirst can lag behind the need for rehydration; thus, water losses should be anticipated and water replaced frequently (every 15 to 20 minutes) in hot environments. In extreme situations with several hours of continuous activity (eg, a marathon), a significant loss of sodium may occur even with water replacement.

Heat rashes are a common problem in hot work environments. Prickly heat is manifested as red papules and usually appears in areas where the clothing is restrictive. As sweating increases, these papules give rise to a prickling sensation. Prickly heat occurs in skin that is persistently wet by unevaporated sweat, and heat rash papules may become infected if they are not treated. In most cases, heat rashes will disappear when the affected individual returns to a cool environment.

A heat stress program helps to minimize the risk of progressive heat stress by promoting situational awareness, ensuring preemptive hydration, setting activity limits based on equipment and environmental conditions, and rehabilitating workers after work cycles.[11,12] Workers should be educated on potential consequences of heat stress, warning signs, and the need for appropriate rest and hydration. Preemptive hydration with 12 to 32 ounces of water reduces the risk of heat-related injury.[11] In hot environments, active work cycles in PPE should be limited to 20 minutes. During rest and rehabilitation cycles, cooling and rehydration are extremely important. Research indicates that active and passive cooling methods produce equivalent reduction in body temperature.[13] Similarly, intravenous and oral rehydration methods produce equivalent cooling.[14] In both of these studies it was noted that cooling, by any method, did not result in a return to baseline temperature during a standard 20-minute rehabilitation period.[13,14] Rehydration can be achieved with water or drinks that contain carbohydrates and/or electrolytes.

Generally, water is the best choice of rehydration solution because of its low cost, wide availability, and lack of complexity. Beverages that contain ethanol or caffeine should be strictly avoided. Drinks with an osmolarity of 270 to 330 mOsm/kg are considered isotonic with blood and extracellular fluids. Drinks that are hypotonic promote fluid absorption, while drinks that are hypertonic inhibit fluid absorption and often cause abdominal pain. In general, it is recommended that rehydration solutions served in rehabilitation not exceed an osmolarity of 350 mOsm/kg. Fruit juices, carbonated sodas, and energy drinks frequently exceed 450 mOsm/kg and would exacerbate dehydration. In some cases commercially available "sports beverages" have osmolarities in excess of 350 mOsm/kg. If such products are used, they should be appropriately diluted with water before serving. Because drink products vary significantly and are frequently reformulated, their use is problematic without significant planning or on-site support from a knowledgeable health care professional. Weight loss during a work cycle can be used as a proxy for fluid loss. Adequacy of rehydration can be assessed by restoration of initial weight and passage of clear urine. An area near by the decontamination site should be established for worker rehabilitation for team members as they rotate. This site should be monitored by medical personnel looking for evidence of heat stress or exhaustion under established protocols. Protocols for return to service should be established; workers should have vital signs within the normal baseline range and should self-assess their ability to continue working.[1,15]

6.6.2   Levels of PPE

Four levels of PPE (levels A, B, C, and D) are defined by OSHA and the US Environmental Protection Agency (Table 6-2).[9,10,15,16] PPE provides an increased level of respiratory and dermal protection. The primary protection needed in a chemical incident response is high-quality respiratory protection. OSHA and the National Institutes for Occupational Safety and Health (NIOSH) have specified respiratory protection levels based on concentrations of chemicals that would be *immediately dangerous to life and health* (IDLH) and *permissible exposure limits* (PELs) for chemicals and radioactive materials. Respirator effectiveness is rated by the fit protection factor, a multiple of the PEL for a specific chemical. For example, if a respirator that has a fit protection factor of 100 is worn and exposed to a contaminant that has a PEL of 1 part

TABLE 6-2 Four Levels of PPE[9,10,15,16]

Level	Equipment	Pros	Cons
Level A	➤ A full facemask with air supplied from a tank or a tether line ➤ Totally encapsulating chemical-protective suit ➤ Gloves and boots are part of suit	➤ Highest level of airway and skin protection	➤ Use limited by supplied air availability ➤ Very hot to work in ➤ Most bulky ➤ Most expensive ➤ Communication is very difficult ➤ Extensive training required
Level B	➤ A full face mask with air supplied from a tank or a tether line ➤ Impermeable, splash- and vapor-resistant suit ➤ Separate or incorporated gloves and boots	➤ Highest level of airway protection ➤ Good skin protection	➤ Use limited by air available ➤ Very hot to work in ➤ Bulky ➤ Expensive ➤ Communication is difficult ➤ Extensive training required
Level C	➤ Masks or hoods (positive or negative pressure) with air filters ➤ Splatter- and vapor-resistant suit ➤ Permeable or impermeable ➤ Separate gloves and boots	➤ Good airway protection ➤ No risk of running out of air ➤ Good skin protection ➤ Less training needed	➤ Filters only protect against specific hazards ➤ Not for use in low oxygen levels ➤ Hot to work in ➤ Bulky ➤ Communication is difficult
Level D	➤ A work uniform affording minimal protection ➤ Universal precautions in a health care facility (gown, hat, mask, face shield, gloves)	➤ No special training needed	➤ No respiratory protection ➤ Limited skin protection

per million (ppm), it will offer protection in an atmosphere with up to 100 ppm or 100 times the PEL.

Fit protection factors vary depending on the respirator. A self-contained breathing apparatus has the highest rating, and negative-pressure air-purifying respirators have the lowest protection ratings.

The next part of PPE is a garment that functions as an effective barrier between harmful materials and the skin. PPE barrier components include gown, gloves, mask, eye protection/face shield, and boots. These are familiar as universal precautions for situations where splash/spray/contact with blood, body fluids, secretions, excretions, mucous membranes, wounds, and contaminated materials can be anticipated.

Levels A and B offer the most protection, but they are cumbersome to use and typically provide less than 1 hour of work time when self-contained air tanks are used. Levels A and B ensembles (Figures 6-5 and 6-6) would be appropriate for entering areas that are known to be heavily contaminated, but they are not necessary for most health care missions. For most chemical decontamination operations in proximity to a hospital, a level C ensemble (Figure 6-7) will be used.[1] Level C equipment consists of a mask or hood with air filters rather than supplied air, and either an impermeable or permeable barrier garment with secured gloves and boots.

Health care workers involved in disaster response may be faced with casualties contaminated by communicable infections, radioactive materials, or chemicals. Each of these different threats requires different types of PPE. Donning is the process of putting on PPE, and doffing is the process of removing PPE. Both should be practiced. The Chapter Appendix provides a checklist for donning and doffing level C PPE.

Safe work practices apply during routine patient and mass casualty care. They reflect hand and body situational awareness:

➤ Keep hands away from face.

➤ Work from clean to dirty.

➤ Limit surfaces touched.

➤ Change garments when torn or heavily contaminated.

➤ Wash hands with soap and water.

Level D PPE is universal precautions in a health care facility. This consists of gown, hat, mask, face shield, and gloves, and may include shoe coverings. Variable skin protection is provided due to the varying permeability of the gown, hat, and mask materials, as well as uncovered areas (eg, partial face, neck, lower legs). Level D PPE with fluid impermeable barrier garments and mask/mask respirators is acceptable for mass casualty events with infectious disease and radioactive contamination. While the concept of universal precautions is simple, the execution of universal precautions is irregular and variable on a daily basis.

6.6.3 PPE for Biologic Casualties

When dealing with biologic casualties, protective equipment requirements are different than those for hazardous material contamination, but the general principles are similar.[3,12,15,17,19] Fluid-impermeable barrier garments and a particulate mask or respirator are needed. For patients with infectious diseases that can be spread by respiratory droplets or are airborne, the risk of transmission is very high. During the 2003 SARS epidemic an estimated 72% of cases were infected in a health care setting and 45% were health care workers.[19] Table 6-3 provides guidelines for reducing transmission of infectious diseases.

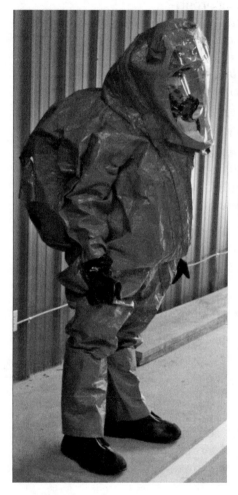
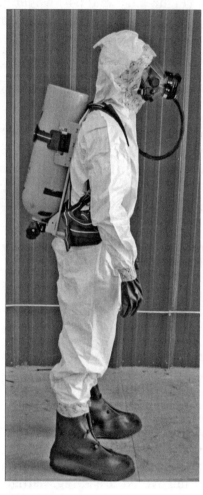
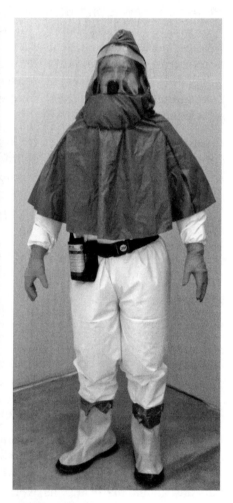

FIGURE 6-5
Example of Level A PPE with Encapsulating Protective Suit and Self-contained Breathing Apparatus

FIGURE 6-6
Example of Level B PPE with Vapor-Protective Suit and Self-contained Breathing Apparatus

FIGURE 6-7
Example of Level C PPE with Splash-Protective Suit and Powered Air-Purifying Respirator

Photos courtesy of Georgia Health Sciences University Department of Emergency Medicine.

TABLE 6-3 Guidelines for Reducing Transmission of Infectious Diseases (adapted from Hostler et al[13])

Precaution	Fluid-Impermeable Gown	Nitrile Gloves	Mask and Eye Cover	Environmental Controls
Standard	Wear if contact with blood or body fluids is expected	Wear if touching blood, body fluids, contaminated items, or mucous membranes	Surgical mask and eye cover should be worn for activities likely to generate splashes or sprays of blood or body fluids	Routine cleaning and disinfection of surfaces
Contact	Wear for all interactions with patient and contaminated environment; don before entering room	Wear for all interactions with patient and contaminated environment; don before entering room	As per standard	Single patient per room preferred; if not possible, consider cohorting
Droplet	As per standard	As per standard	Don surgical mask on entering room; eye cover per standard	As above plus use of curtains; patient should wear mask when out of room
Airborne	As per standard	As per standard	Wear fit-tested N95 respirator or powered air-purifying respirator when entering patient room	Place patient in negative-pressure isolation room with 6–12 air exchanges/h

Donning PPE for Universal Precautions

PPE should be put on in the following order before entering the patient's room.

1. Gown

➤ Fully cover torso from neck to knees, arms to end of wrist, and wrap around back.

➤ Fasten back at neck and waist.

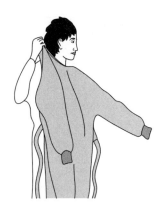
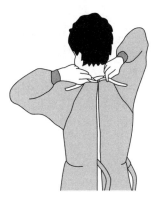

2. Mask or respirator

➤ Secure ties or elastic band at middle of head and neck.

➤ Fit flexible band to nose bridge.

➤ Fit snug to face and below chin.

➤ Fit-check respirator.

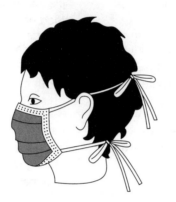 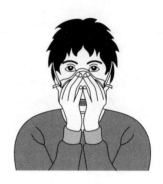

3. Goggles or face shield

➤ Put on face and adjust to fit.

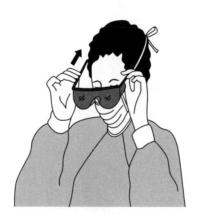 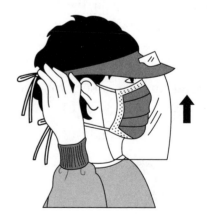

4. Gloves

➤ Use nonsterile for isolation.

➤ Select according to hand size.

➤ Extend to cover wrist of isolation gown.

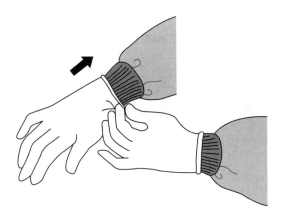

Doffing PPE for Universal Precautions

PPE should be removed in the following order at the exit of the contaminated space.

1. Gloves

➤ Outside of gloves is contaminated.

➤ Grasp outside of glove with opposite gloved hand; peel off.

➤ Hold removed glove in gloved hand.

➤ Slide fingers of ungloved hand under remaining glove at wrist; peel off.

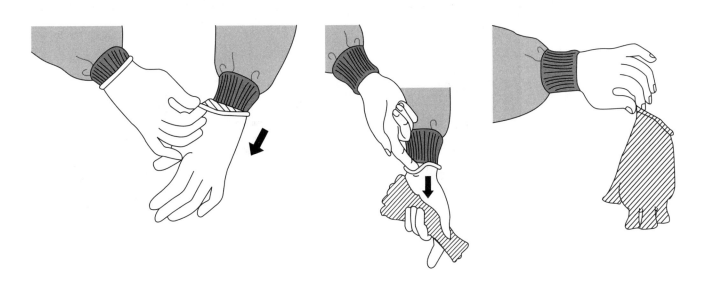

2. Goggles/face shield

➤ Outside of goggles or face shield is contaminated.

➤ To remove, handle by "clean" headband or ear pieces.

➤ Place in designated receptacle for reprocessing or in waste container.

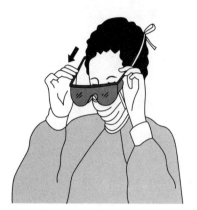 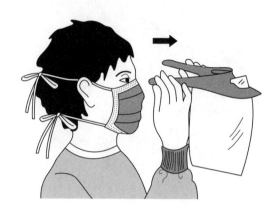

3. Gown

➤ Gown front and sleeves are contaminated.

➤ Unfasten neck, then waist ties.

➤ Remove gown in a peeling motion; pull gown from shoulder toward the hand.

➤ Gown will turn inside out.

➤ Hold removed gown away from body, roll into a bundle and discard into an appropriate receptacle.

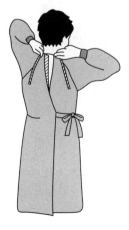 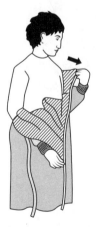 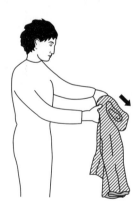

4. Mask or respirator

➤ Front of mask/respirator is contaminated; do not touch.

➤ Grasp *only* bottom, then top ties/elastics, and remove.

➤ Discard in waste container.

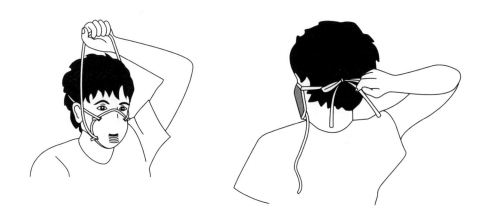

5. Hand Hygiene

➤ Wash hands immediately after removing all PPE.

6.6.4   PPE for Radioactive Contamination

The main need for PPE when dealing with low-level radioactive contamination is to keep the airway, skin, and personal clothing free of droplet or particulate contaminants.[4] Waterproof barrier garments will effectively limit radioactive energy from alpha particles and beta particles, but not gamma rays. After a radiation event, brief exposure to radioactive energy that may penetrate garments is of little risk to the worker.[4,20] The major risk is becoming contaminated by a *source* of radiation and then receiving a larger ongoing exposure over time.[4,20] Hence, it is more important for protective garments to prevent contamination than to shield against radiation. Thicker garments are preferred over lead aprons, which impair movement and offer similar protection.[4]

Radiological PPE is similar to what is used for biologic contamination, with the addition of waterproof shoe and head covers, as well as taping of all seams and cuffs.[4] Two pairs of surgical gloves should be worn. The first pair (inner glove) should go under the arm cuff and be secured by tape. The second pair (outer glove) is worn over and not taped. A radiation dosimeter should be assigned to each team member and attached to the outside of the surgical gown at the neck. Gloves should be checked for contamination with a survey meter periodically to limit transfer or spread of radioactive contamination.

Components of Level C PPE[1]

➤ A powered air-purifying respirator with a protection factor of 1000.

➤ A NIOSH-approved respirator with combination 99.97% high-efficiency particulate air (HEPA)/ organic vapor/acid gas respirator cartridges.

➤ Double- or triple-layer protective gloves.

➤ Chemical-resistant suit with head covering and eye/face protection (if not part of the respirator).

➤ Chemical-protective boots.

➤ Tape-sealed interfaces (eg, suit/boots, suit/gloves).

Donning and doffing procedures are essentially the same as for biologic contamination, with an additional step for workers to be checked for contamination with a survey meter after removal of garments.

6.6.5   PPE for Chemical Contamination

Chemical PPE should offer both respiratory and dermal protection.[1,2] When responding to casualties with chemical contamination in situations where the contaminant is unknown, or gross contamination and clinical symptoms are seen, level C PPE is appropriate for workers performing decontamination adjacent to health care facilities.[1]

A powered air-purifying respirator (PAPR) is a filtering device that stops particulate matter and chemically adsorbs or neutralizes selected toxins that are too small to filter. The optimal garment material for first receivers will protect against a wide range of chemicals in liquid, solid, or vapor form, yet also be sufficiently flexible, durable, and lightweight during physically active work. Protection from gases is less important because gases generally will dissipate before a casualty arrives at the hospital. OSHA sets standard for PPE manufacturers but does not test or endorse specific products. Manufacturers produce a variety of suit designs and perform testing of chemical breakthrough times. Several suit fabrics may be appropriate, depending on the situations and hazards that health care workers may encounter.[1,7] Some have hoods and/or feet, while others do not. The suit selected should be compatible with the required respirator. The ability of protective garment fabric to withstand physical abrasion and tearing is also important. Before materials are selected, the manufacturer should be contacted for guidance and laboratory-testing information regarding specific materials should be obtained and reviewed.

No single glove or boot material will protect against every substance. Manufacturers offer detailed guides to materials and their chemical resistance. Butyl rubber gloves generally provide better protection than nitrile gloves for chemical warfare agents and most toxic industrial chemicals that are more likely to be involved in a terrorist incident, although the converse applies to some industrial chemicals. Foil-based gloves are highly resistant to a wide variety of hazardous substances and could also be considered when determining an appropriate protective ensemble. Hospitals must select gloves that cover the specific substances that the hospital has determined first receivers reasonably might encounter. However, given the broad scope of potential contaminants, OSHA considers it of vital importance for hospitals also to select materials that protect against a wide range of substances.[1] A double layer of gloves, made of two different materials, or foil-based gloves protect against the broadest range of chemicals.

For example, a combination of butyl gloves worn over inner nitrile gloves is often the best option for use by hospital workers during emergencies and mass casualties involving hazardous substances. Glove thickness is measured in mils, with a higher number of mils indicating a thicker glove. Using common examples, examination gloves are 4 mil, while general-purpose household (kitchen) gloves are 12 to 16 mil, and heavy industrial gloves are 20 to 30 mil. Note that thinner gloves deteriorate (tear and rip) more rapidly than thicker gloves. When thinner gloves must be used, they should be changed frequently. Depending on the dexterity needed by the hospital worker, the glove selection can be modified to allow for the use of a glove combination that is thinner than that usually recommended for the best protection. In general, the same material selected for gloves will also be appropriate for boots. Because boot walls tend to be thicker than gloves, boots of any material are likely to be more protective than gloves of the same material.

Examples of Tested Protective Suits and Protection Factor Against Vapors[21]

➤ Tyvek Protective Wear Suit: 4x greater than nothing.

➤ Tychem 9400 Protective Suit: 17x greater than nothing.

➤ Tychem SL Protective Suit: 24x greater than nothing.

➤ Tyvek ProTech F Protective: 42x greater than nothing.

6.7 SUMMARY

Worker safety in disaster response cannot be overemphasized; not only are injured workers unable to perform the response mission, they add to the casualty load.

The process of decontamination and the prevention of worker contamination through PPE entail heavy logistics. To be effective when needed, decontamination and wearing of PPE should be practiced at regular intervals. Though this chapter has emphasized decontamination and wearing of PPE under ideal conditions, their application in a real mass casualty situation will add significantly to the complexity of the response.

REFERENCES

1. Occupational Safety and Health Administration. OSHA best practices for hospital-based first receivers of victims from mass casualty incidents involving the release of hazardous substances. January 2005. http://www.osha.gov/dts/osta/bestpractices/firstreceivers_hospital.pdf Accessed July 30, 2011.

2. US Army and Soldier and Biological Chemical Command (SBCCOM). Guidelines for mass casualty decontamination during a terrorist chemical agent incident. January 2000. http://www.chem-bio.com/resource/2000/cwirp_guidelines_mass.pdf. Accessed July 30, 2011.

3. Siegel JD, Rhinehart E, Jackson M, Chiarello L, Healthcare Infection Control Practices Advisory Committee. 2007 Guideline for Isolation Precautions: Preventing Transmission of Infectious Agents in Healthcare Settings. June 2007. http://www.cdc.gov/hicpac/pdf/isolation/Isolation2007.pdf. Accessed February 20, 2011.

4. Smith JM, Spano MA. CDC Interim Guidelines for Hospital Response to Mass Casualties from a Radiological Incident. December 2003. http://www.bt.cdc.gov/radiation/pdf/MassCasualtiesGuidelines.pdf.

5. Subbarao I, Lyznicki J, Hsu E, et.al., A Consensus-based Educational Framework and Competency Set for the Discipline of Disaster Medicine and Public Health Preparedness. *Disaster Med Public Health Prep.* 2008;2:57–68.

6. Feldman RJ. Chemical agent simulant release from clothing following vapor exposure. *Acad Emerg Med.* 2010;17(2):221–224.

7. Okumura T, Takasu N, Ishimatsu S, et al. Report on 640 victims of the Tokyo subway sarin attack. *Ann Emerg Med.* 1996;28(2):129–135.

8. US Army Soldier and Biological Chemical Command (SBCCOM). Guidelines for cold weather mass decontamination during a chemical agent incident. January 2002; revised August 2003. http://www.ecbc.army.mil/downloads/cwirp/ECBC_cwirp_cold_weather_mass_decon.pdf.

9. OSHA respiratory standards 29.1910.134. Code of Federal Register. http://www.osha.gov/pls/oshaweb/owadisp.show_document?p_table=STANDARDS&p_id=12716. Accessed October 25, 2009.

10. HAZWOPER standards 29.1910.120 Code of Federal Register. http://www.osha.gov/pls/oshaweb/owadisp.show_document?p_table=STANDARDS&p_id=9765. Accessed October 25, 2009.

11. US Fire Administration. Emergency Incident Rehabilitation. February 2008. http://www.usfa.dhs.gov/downloads/pdf/publications/fa_314.pdf.

12. Heubner KD, Lavonas E, Arnold JL. CBRNE – personal protective equipment. *eMedicine.* June 2009. http://emedicine.medscape.com/article/831240-overview.

13. Hostler D, Reis SE, Bednez JC, Kerin S, Suyama J. Comparison of active cooling devices with passive cooling for rehabilitation of firefighters performing exercise in thermal protective clothing: a report from the Fireground Rehab Evaluation (FIRE) Trial. *Prehospital Emerg Care.* 2010;14(3):300-309.

14. Hostler D, Bednez JC, Kerin S, et al. Comparison of rehydration regimens for rehabilitation of firefighters performing heavy exercise in thermal protective clothing: a report from the Fireground Rehab Evaluation (FIRE) Trial. *Prehospital Emerg Care.* 2010;14(2):194–201.

15. OSHA personal protective equipment standards 29.1910.132. Code of Federal Register. http://www.osha.gov/pls/oshaweb/owadisp.show_document?p_table=STANDARDS&p_id=9777. Accessed October 25, 2009.

16. HAZWOPER standards Appendix B 29.1910.120. Code of Federal Register. http://www.osha.gov/pls/oshaweb/owadisp.show_document?p_table=STANDARDS&p_id=9767. Accessed October 25, 2009.

17. Bolyard EA, Tablan OC, Williams WW, et al. Guideline for infection control in health care personnel, 1998. *Am J Infect Control.* 1998;26:289–354.

18. Daugherty E. Health care worker protection in mass casualty respiratory failure: infection control, decontamination, and personal protective equipment. *Respiratory Care.* 2008;53(2):201–214.

19. Centers for Disease Control and Prevention. Cluster of severe acute respiratory syndrome cases among protected health-care workers—Toronto, Canada, April 2003. *MMWR Morb Mortal Wkly Rep.* 2003;52(19):433–436.

20. International Atomic Energy Agency. Manual for First Responders to a Radiological Emergency. October 2006. http://www.pub.iaea.org/MTCD/publications/PDF/EPR_FirstResponder_web.pdf.

21. US Army Soldier and Biological Command. Guidelines for use of personal protective equipment by law enforcement personnel during a terrorist chemical agent incident. June 2001; revised December 2003. http://www.edgewood.army.mil/downloads/cwirp/ECBC_ppe_law_enforcement_ca_incident.pdf.

APPENDIX LEVEL C PPE DONNING AND DOFFING PROCEDURES CHECKLIST

Donning

Assumptions

Suit features

➤ Booties attached

➤ Hood

➤ Front entry

Assistant helping

Preparation Steps

Hydrate

Remove sharp objects

Remove personnel items (watch, wallet, etc)

Donning Steps

1. Leave shoes on

2. Don suit to waist

3. Attach paper clip to zipper

4. Sit down

5. Pre-event medical monitoring

6. Don booties (1 of 2 types: tight or loose fitting)

7. Tape boot to suit (leg raised/add tab)

8. Don inner gloves

9. Don outer (chemical-resistant) gloves

10. Place arms into suit (placing suit wrist area on top of glove)*

11. Place arms into a position of function

12. Tape gloves to suit (add tab)

13. Stand up, place PAPR belt on waist

14. Turn on PAPR unit

15. Don PAPR hood

Applies only to working with hands pointing down. Reverse for above-the-head work.

16. Tuck in inner segment of PAPR hood

17. Zip up

18. Seal or tape zipper or storm flap (18" with tab on center back/belt height, bring up to front between legs)

   a. Tape is not required if suit has a self-sealing storm flap

19. Don additional gloves as needed (anticontamination or sizing issue)

20. Place name tape on thigh or back of hood

21. Place triage tape on forearm (optional)

Doffing Steps

Assumptions

Assistant helping

Preparation Steps

Exit contaminated area

Process through decontamination

Doffing Steps

1. Remove ALL tape from booties

2. Remove tape from zipper seam

3. Remove overgloves

4. Remove tape from wrists

5. Remove booties

6. Detach PAPR belt

7. Support PAPR (assistant or chair)

8. Zip suit down all the way

9. Pull suit down to ankles

10. Wearer sits down (on clean chair)

11. Remove suit (step into cold zone one leg at a time)

12. Remove outer gloves (keep inner gloves on)

13. Remove PAPR hood

14. Remove inner gloves

15. Exit undressing area

Check vitals and replace water

CHAPTER | SEVEN

Mass Casualty Management

Frederick L. Slone, MD

John H. Armstrong, MD

7.1 PURPOSE

This chapter reviews mass casualty clinical management in the context of specific mechanisms of disaster.

7.2 LEARNING OBJECTIVES

After completing this chapter, learners will be able to:

➤ Demonstrate clinical casualty evaluation and management appropriate to the context of mass casualties in simulated all-hazards events.

➤ Apply life-saving interventions on a simulated casualty.

➤ Differentiate clinical care delivered in a mass casualty environment from usual clinical practice.

7.3 DISASTER MEDICINE AND PUBLIC HEALTH PREPAREDNESS COMPETENCIES ADDRESSED

➤ Access timely and credible health and safety information for all ages and populations affected by natural disasters, industrial- or transportation-related catastrophes (eg, hazardous material spill, explosion), epidemics, and acts of terrorism (eg, involving conventional and nuclear explosives and/or release of biologic, chemical, and radiologic agents). (2.2.4)

➤ Demonstrate the ability to apply and adapt clinical knowledge and skills for the assessment and management of injuries and illnesses in victims of all ages under various exposure scenarios (eg, natural disasters, industrial- or transportation-related catastrophes; epidemics; and acts of terrorism involving conventional and nuclear explosives and/or release of biologic, chemical, and radiological agents), in accordance with professional scope of practice. (5.2.3)

7.4 INTRODUCTION

"Imagination is more important than knowledge. For knowledge is limited to all we now know and understand, while imagination embraces the entire world, and all there ever will be to know and understand." Einstein's assertion resonates when the management of the "mass" in mass casualties is considered. To shift from usual clinical thinking focused on the individual patient to a disaster mindset focused on the casualty population requires imagination. Uncertainty is the rule. When the casualties become apparent, multiple variables remain unknown, including casualty number, resource availability, and event duration. "More business, managed as usual" thinking in a mass casualty situation substitutes accessible familiarity for needed creativity and lessens the outcome for the casualty population.

7.5 MECHANISMS OF DISASTER

Casualties are generated by mechanisms of disaster that are beyond routine experience: explosions, incendiaries, and dissemination of chemical, radiological, and biologic agents. Specific clinical presentations are unfamiliar to daily clinical practice and may include multidimensional blast injuries; crush syndromes, multicompartment syndromes, and traumatic asphyxiation; nerve, blood, pulmonary, and vesicant agents; radiation; and class A biologic agents. Successful management of an individual casualty from these mechanisms requires application of different care paradigms and skills. Yet preparation involves more than understanding the care of an individual disaster casualty under ideal circumstances; it entails the integration of care across a casualty population under disaster conditions.

Disaster mechanisms define the nature of casualty management. While many events occur with a single disaster mechanism, some have multiple primary and secondary ("second hit") mechanisms. It is important to think with imagination about nonobvious associated mechanisms, either synchronous or metachronous with the obvious mechanism.

Casualties with physical trauma reflect physical events, whether explosions, structural collapse, mass gunfire, or incendiaries. While physical trauma from an explosion is apparent, there may be more to the story. Casualties presenting with acute hearing loss may be manifesting exposure to high-energy explosions. Explosions may be simultaneous or sequential, as well as intentional (eg, terrorism) or unintentional (eg, exposed utilities). The initial blast mechanisms may be followed by major crush injury due to structural collapse, electrocution from bare electrical wires, or exposure to smoke and gases as byproducts of combustion. A "dirty bomb" event combines a conventional explosive with radioactive material, which may elude detection when the possibility is not considered. A nuclear event is the ultimate explosion, which includes blast injuries and radiation.

Radiation casualties can present with emerging burns and acute radiation syndromes. The former may not be evident for several days, and the latter can be predicted clinically by the timeline from the event of casualty emesis. With increasing radiation exposure, progressive hematopoietic, gastrointestinal, and neurovascular syndromes appear.[1]

Casualties from chemical and biologic agents present with illness, rather than injury, and can be differentiated by considering the timeline and geography of presentation. Chemical events produce casualties at the same time, in the same area, and from the exposed area simultaneously. Biologic events, on the other hand, tend to occur with scattered groups of casualties who present over a longer period to multiple hospitals across a wider geography. Containment of a chemical event is challenging in the acute interval, whereas control of a biologic event is very demanding over the subacute period. After the general classification of illness, the particular agent responsible for chemical or biologic event requires further determination. Analyzing casualty population symptoms and signs as a constellation enables more rapid navigation to the mechanism of illness.

7.6 SAFETY AND HAZARDS

Appropriate personal protective equipment (PPE) for first responders and health care receivers must be matched to the suspected agent to prevent exposure to and spread of the agent. The worst-case scenario must be considered with imagination. Without consideration of potential contamination, first responders and receivers can become contaminated casualties, thus increasing the number of casualties while simultaneously reducing resources. A higher level of PPE is usually required at the scene than at a health care facility because of uncertainty regarding the source coupled with the concentrated contamination at the scene (see Chapter 6). PPE used at the health care facility according to the disaster mechanism is described in Figure 7-1.[2]

Myths abound regarding PPE and radioactive agents. To define what PPE is needed for radiologic events, one must differentiate between exposure and contamination. A casualty who was exposed to radiation is *not* radioactive and does not pose any risk to others; the casualty may have radiation injury, but there is no residual radioactivity due to radiation exposure. On the other hand, a casualty who is contaminated with *radioactive material* may pose a small risk to the health care provider: the source of radioactivity is on the casualty and, depending on its location (eg, skin, wounds), may be exposing the casualty to ongoing radiation. Casualty decontamination (see below) is necessary to remove any ongoing radiation exposure for the casualty and to limit the spread of contamination to the uninjured, including health care providers. Universal precautions

FIGURE 7-1
PPE at Health Care Facility
According to Mechanism

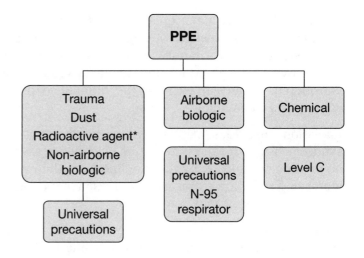

*Consider aerosolized nature of radioactive debris, with added benefit of N-95 mask respirator.

provide an effective barrier for radiation from alpha (plutonium, radium, uranium) and beta (cobalt, iodine) particles, which are both relatively nonpenetrating (clothing prevents penetration). Radioactive dust or debris can be inhaled or ingested, leading to internal contamination; a standard surgical mask affords adequate protection, though an N-95 mask is recommended if available. In the hospital setting, the amount of contamination on any one casualty will likely be so minimal that an N-95 mask will not add to protection.[3] Gamma radiation is wave radiation (ie, not particulate) that results from a nuclear reaction; it is not a source of contamination on a casualty.[4]

Decontamination of mass casualties is very difficult. Assumptions about ideal casualty behavior, such as orderly lines, are invalid, and the logistics are significant. Each step escalates the subsequent logistical requirements for the casualty population (eg, disposition of contaminated clothing; towels and cover for wet, naked casualties). The decontamination literature tends to focus on the ideal single or multiple contaminated casualty event, rather than mass contaminated casualties. Simplicity is paramount for successful mass decontamination. Casualty decontamination can be readily accomplished by dry (removing clothes) and wet (washing with soap and water) methods (Figure 7-2).[5] Focus areas for wet decontamination include wounds, hair, and skin creases/folds. Radioactive debris should be treated like dirt with dry and wet decontamination. Planning based on sufficient reactive decontaminants for nerve or vesicant agents is based on the flawed notion that these countermeasures are readily available; they are typically not available in timely (minutes to hours, respectively) fashion.

Decontamination must be considered adjacent to the scene and outside of health care facilities. Assuming casualty decontamination at the scene is inconsistent with the evidence that most casualties self-transport from the scene to health care facilities. Decontamination in a health care facility renders the health care facility contaminated; instead, it should occur away from the primary casualty triage point and hospital entry.[6]

FIGURE 7-2
Decontamination Algorithm

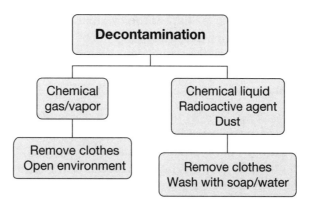

7.7 CLINICAL PRESENTATION AND MANAGEMENT OF EXPLOSION INJURIES

Blast injury has four potential components: primary (overpressure), secondary (penetrating), tertiary (blunt, impalement), and quaternary (burns, crush, contamination, exacerbations of preexisting illnesses). Though the injury presentations are grouped within blast components below, the real challenge is managing casualties with combinations of these blast injuries. Such multi-dimensional injuries represent a mix of traumatic mechanisms of injury in a single casualty.

7.7.1 Primary Effects

Pulmonary blast injury (PBI) should be suspected in anyone with dyspnea, cough, hemoptysis, or chest pain after blast exposure. Blast lung injury behaves like severe pulmonary contusion with progressive hypoxia. Signs of blast lung injury are usually present at the time of initial evaluation, but they have been reported as late as 48 hours after the explosion. Supplemental oxygen, judicious fluid resuscitation, and supportive ventilator care are the mainstays of treatment. Airway pressures should be kept as low as possible, while still maintaining adequate oxygenation and ventilation, to limit arterial gas embolism.[7]

Tension pneumothorax may result from abrupt rupture of visceral pleura due to the blast pressure wave (or due to penetrating trauma [secondary] or blunt force trauma with rib fractures [tertiary]). This leads to air in the chest cavity under pressure. Tension pneumothorax presents with severe respiratory distress, absent or diminished breath sounds on the affected side, distended neck veins, and hypotension. The treatment of a tension pneumothorax is needle decompression (see Appendix). Needle decompression converts an emergent issue into an urgent one, then requiring chest tube placement.[8]

Arterial gas embolism is a consequence of PBI. Air emboli result from a direct communication between disrupted pulmonary vasculature and the bronchial tree. More air will enter the circulation whenever venous pressure is lower than bronchial airway pressure. Therefore, air emboli may follow intubation and positive-pressure ventilation. Air embolism is believed to be responsible for most of the sudden deaths within the first hour after blast exposure. In mass casualty management, suspicion of air embolism is an expectant consideration.[8]

Blast auditory injury is marked by acute hearing loss at time of presentation. Other signs include tinnitus, otalgia, vertigo, and bleeding from the external auditory canal. Tympanic membrane perforation is the most common injury of the middle ear. If tympanic membrane rupture has occurred or is likely to have occurred, any irrigation or probing of the ear canal should be avoided.[9] There is *no* consistent correlation between tympanic membrane perforation and other blast injuries.[10]

Blast abdominal injury includes perforations of the gastrointestinal tract (most likely the cecum) and mesenteric devascularization. Blast abdominal injury should be suspected in anyone exposed to an explosion who has abdominal pain, nausea, vomiting, or hematemesis. Guarding and rebound tenderness may be present. Clinical findings may be absent initially and may take hours to progress. If bowel perforation or mesenteric ischemia is suspected, surgical intervention will be needed. Otherwise, these casualties are in the delayed category and require interval reevaluations.[8]

7.7.2   Secondary and Tertiary Effects

Secondary injuries may be related to explosive fragments that penetrate visceral compartments or lacerate vessels. Hemorrhage may be significant. Ocular globe injuries may occur as well; eye examination is relevant later in the sequence of care. Tertiary injuries result from the blast wind that throws casualties in the air, with blunt force trauma or impalement on objects occurring when the casualties hit ground. Traumatic amputation may occur as well. Open wounds should be managed by stopping the bleeding with direct pressure. They subsequently require copious irrigation and debridement; as dirty wounds, they should *not* be closed primarily. Tetanus toxoid and therapeutic antibiotics are appropriate. Impaled objects should not be removed from casualties; rather, such objects should be stabilized on the casualty and removed subsequently in a controlled setting (ie, an operating room) by a surgeon.[8]

Traumatic amputation of any limb is a marker for multisystem injuries. Bleeding from mangled extremities and traumatic amputations can normally be controlled with tourniquets; in a mass casualty situation, the use of tourniquets can increase the greatest good for the greatest number. Tourniquets are inexpensive, easily applied, and extremely effective to stop bleeding from an extremity. Although the application of the tourniquet for more than 6 hours may be associated with distal tissue loss, allowing an extremity to bleed uncontrollably will lead to early loss of life.[11] Appropriate use of tourniquets in a system of mass casualty response requires the use of a standardized protocol that links prehospital and hospital use (see Appendix).

7.7.3 Quaternary Effects

Crush injury results from extremity or torso compressions that cause direct tissue injury and tissue ischemia. Typically affected areas of the body include lower extremities (74%), upper extremities (10%), and trunk (9%).[12]

Crush syndrome is localized crush injury with systemic manifestations. These systemic effects are caused by traumatic rhabdomyolysis (muscle breakdown) and the release of potentially toxic muscle cell components and electrolytes into the circulatory system. Profound acidemia, hyperkalemia, and hyperphosphatemia, coupled with organ dysfunction, result. Sudden release of crushed, trapped extremities results in acute reperfusion and profound crush syndrome. Management includes, when possible, preemptive application of tourniquets on crushed extremities to limit acute reperfusion and crush syndrome. This is followed by volume expansion with intravenous (IV) normal saline; lactated Ringer's solution has potassium and should be avoided in this situation. The infusion rate should be 1 to 1.5 L/h, with an ultimate urine output goal of 200 to 300 mL/h until myoglobinuria has ceased. Alkalinization of the urine to help prevent myoglobin precipitation in the renal tubules may be helpful; this is accomplished by administering sequential ampules of sodium bicarbonate until the urine pH is greater than 6.5. Hyperkalemia should be anticipated and can be lethal. Calcium, though cardioprotective in other settings of hyperkalemia, may enable calcium phosphate precipitation in the setting of hyperphosphatemia due to crush syndrome. If electrocardiographic (ECG) signs of hypocalcemia develop, with widening of the QRS complex or loss of p waves, then 10 mL of 10% calcium gluconate or 5 mL of 10% calcium chloride should be given IV over 2 minutes.

Hyperkalemia can be identified with rapid point-of-care testing and monitored with an ECG rhythm strip. It requires rapid intervention based on suggestive ECG changes (tall, peaked T waves with a shortened Q-T interval). Initial treatment consists of movement of serum potassium intracellularly with 10 units of regular insulin IV followed by one ampule of D50, then one ampule of sodium bicarbonate (45 mEq) IV over 5 minutes, repeated in 30 minutes. When available, albuterol can also move potassium into cells; it can be administered via nebulizer, 10 to 20 mg in 4 mL of saline, over 10 minutes, or IV, 0.5 mg. Insulin and glucose, bicarbonate, and albuterol are only temporizing measures for management of life-threatening hyperkalemia; ultimately, potassium needs to be removed via the gastrointestinal tract with a potassium-binding resin (Kaexylate, 25–50 g, in 100 mL of 20% sorbitol, orally or per rectum) or via the bloodstream with hemodialysis.

Experience with crush injuries from structural collapse in earthquakes indicates a 2% to 15% incidence of crush syndrome; 50% of those with crush syndrome develop acute renal failure, with half of these needing dialysis.[13] Management of casualties with crush syndrome is resource intense.

Extremity compartment syndrome is a result of increased pressure within the fascial compartments of an extremity, leading to neurovascular and organ compromise. Tissue swelling within the compartment results from compression injury or reperfusion of ischemic tissues. Though it is often taught to be recognized by the six *p*'s (pain, pallor, poikilothermia, pulselessness, paresthesias, and paralysis), the last five signs lead to irreversible injury. The earliest sign of compartment syndrome is severe extremity pain in the lucid casualty. In the leg, calf tenderness, bruising, and swelling may also be seen. Distal pulses may still be present in emerging compartment syndrome. When a leg compartment syndrome is evolving, four-compartment fasciotomy (surgical incisions made through the fascia surrounding the compartment) should be performed as soon as possible by a qualified provider. Irreversible muscle damage may occur within 6 hours, with irreversible nerve damage occurring sooner.[8]

Traumatic asphyxia occurs when the chest is compressed by a heavy object to such a degree that blood flow into the thorax and respirations are impeded. Children are somewhat more vulnerable than adults due to their relatively more pliable and cartilaginous chest wall. The marked increase in thoracic pressure causes the blood to back up through the superior vena cava into the veins of the head and neck. Signs and symptoms include respiratory distress, chest ecchymoses (bruising), facial plethora, and subconjunctival hemorrhages. Cerebral hypoxia may lead to altered mental status, seizures, or coma. Rapid extrication with release from compression is the single most important factor in improved survival. Control of the airway, supplemental oxygen, and ventilator support follow. Associated torso injuries, including hemopneumothorax, rib fractures, and pelvic fractures, must be identified.[14]

Burns can be severe and average more than 50% total body surface area (TBSA). Initial management focuses on sustainment of airway and breathing, volume resuscitation, and normothermia. Hyperdynamic physiology and wound consequences emerge after 24 hours, so that mass burn casualty management is permissive (ie, tolerant of essential physiologic management without more advanced burn wound care) for the first 24 hours. Whereas daily practice would promote transfer of a patient with 50% TBSA burns to a burn center immediately, this may not be possible in a burn mass casualty; permissiveness for the first 24 hours permits phased casualty transfer. Any hospital should be prepared to manage a burn patient for the first 24 hours.[15]

7.8 CLINICAL PRESENTATION AND MANAGEMENT OF CHEMICAL AGENT TOXICITIES

Nerve agents: The clinical presentation of casualties from nerve agents is wet, wet, wet—diarrhea, urination, miosis (small pupils), bronchorrhea, bronchospasm, emesis, lacrimation, and salivation (DUMBBELS). Another mnemonic is SLUDGEM (salivation, lacrimation, urination, defecation, gastrointestinal upset, emesis, and miosis). Although miosis and bradycardia (slow heart rate) are often associated with nerve agents, they are not invariably present and are not reliable indicators of a nerve agent.

Atropine and pralidoxime chloride are used to treat nerve agent exposure. The DuoDote kit consists of a single auto-injector cartridge that contains both 2 mg of atropine and 600 mg of pralidoxime chloride (see Appendix). Atropine is used to quickly reverse the cholinergic effects of the nerve agent; sequential doses of atropine, 2 mg IV or intramuscularly (IM) are titrated to relief of respiratory distress and clearing of bronchial secretions. Next, pralidoxime chloride is given (600 mg to 1 g IM or slow IV over 20–30 minutes) to reactivate the acetylcholinesterase enzyme that the nerve agent inhibits. Diazepam is given as well (usually 5–10 mg IV or IM) to treat seizures. A Mark I auto-injector kit consists of 2 auto-injector pens: one pen has 2 mg of atropine and the other has 600 mg of pralidoxime chloride (see Appendix 1).[16] It is anticipated that because of easier use, the single auto-injector cartridge (DuoDote kit) will replace the double injector cartridge (Mark I) over time.

Cyanide agents: These are cyanide compounds and present with rapid onset of symptoms in seconds to minutes—dizziness, weakness, headache, nausea or vomiting with chest tightness, shortness of breath, and profound air hunger—and progress to seizures and coma. The most important steps in treatment are to move the casualties away from the cyanide exposure and administer 100% oxygen.[5] In a true mass casualty situation, the standard regimens for individual patients with cyanide poisoning (hydroxocobalamin or amyl nitrite–sodium nitrite– sodium thiosulfate) will likely have little utility due to limited availability.

Pulmonary agents: Presentation varies with the solubility of the specific gas. Intact skin is not affected.

More water-soluble agents, such as ammonia, hydrogen chloride, formaldehyde, and sulfur dioxide, cause burning of the eyes and mucous membranes of the nose, mouth, and throat, tearing, coughing, and severe throat irritation. Most of the effects are at or above the level of the vocal cords; laryngospasm is a significant concern. Ammonia is easily recognized by its noxious smell, yet smell remains unreliable in general for hazard identification. When a smell is present, the concern should be responder safety.[17]

Moderately water-soluble agents, such as chlorine, also cause burning of the eyes, nose, mouth, and throat, yet cause bronchiole irritation producing bronchospasm and wheezing as well. Chlorine gas has an easily recognized and characteristic bleach smell.[17]

Poorly water-soluble agents, such as phosgene, descend into the alveoli, with minimal eye and upper airway irritation. However, after several hours (and up to 24 hours), symptoms may progress through chest pain to severe respiratory distress and noncardiogenic pulmonary edema with severe shortness of breath and frothy sputum. Phosgene is reported to have the smell of newly mown grass or hay.[17]

Supportive care is the mainstay of treatment, and there are significant logistical issues, particularly as mechanical ventilation is needed for a large number of casualties. With phosgene, IV corticosteroids may be considered to help reduce subsequent inflammation.

Vesicant agents: These are sulfur mustard and lewisite. Both cause burning of the eyes, nose, and throat with tearing, rhinorrhea, cough, and shortness of breath, accompanied by skin blistering with a deep burning sensation. Symptoms start within minutes of lewisite exposure, while symptoms of sulfur mustard exposure start within hours. A specific antidote for lewisite is British anti-lewisite (BAL) agent, also known as dimercaprol. This is a chelating agent that binds to the arsenic molecule of lewisite. It should be used only in patients with shock or severe pulmonary injury because BAL itself can have severe side effects. For sulfur mustard, there is no specific antidote, and supportive care is the only management strategy. For both agents, pain control is imperative.[14]

Rapid differentiation of the specific chemical agent rests with considering dominant symptoms and signs, as outlined in Table 7-1. Events with nerve, blood, and pulmonary agents have two casualty peaks: mass fatalities at the scene and exposed walking wounded.

7.9 CLINICAL PRESENTATION AND MANAGEMENT OF RADIATION INJURY

Radiation causes a wide range of symptoms, depending on the total dose received. The most immediate symptoms are "prodromal" and related to gastric distress. Time to first emesis is a useful triage tool: casualties who vomit within 1 hour of exposure have received lethal radiation and are expectant. If emesis occurs after 4 hours, such casualties are delayed, with high survival rates. Between 1 to 4 hours, casualties are classified as immediate in terms of radiation injury, and survival probability is intermediate. Casualty management is supportive.[4] Radiation burns are managed like thermal burns, yet the challenge with radiation burns is significantly delayed wound healing. Associated traumatic injuries in a radiation casualty require rapid operation and wound closure; radiation injury to the immune system (responsible for wound healing) limits intervention for wounds between days 3 and 60.[1]

There are several specific chelating agents available to help reduce the injury from radioactive agents. The practical problem is that these are radionuclide-specific and must be administered rapidly to be effective.[18] For completeness, the agents

TABLE 7-1 Differentiation of Chemical and Radiation Casualties[4,5]

Symptoms and Signs	Nerve Agents	Blood Agents	Pulmonary Agents	Mustard Agents	Radiation
Vomiting	XX	XX	X (phosgene)		XX
Secretions	XX				
Pinpoint pupils	XX				
Convulsions	XX	XX			
Tachypnea		XX	X	X	
Odor		XX	XX	XX	
Dry cough, wheezing			XX	X	
Blisters				XX	
Burns					XX

X's indicate degree of symptom/sign expression.

are listed in Table 7-2, but the practical utility of these agents in a mass casualty exposure, in adult or pediatric care, is very limited. It is difficult to administer mass chelating agents within the appropriate interval after exposure.

7.10 CLINICAL PRESENTATION AND MANAGEMENT OF CATEGORY A BIOLOGIC AGENT INFECTIONS

Category A biologic agents pose the highest population and casualty risk due to ease of transmissibility, mortality risk, and resource requirements.

Anthrax: Inhalational anthrax has a septic presentation with fever, respiratory distress, shock, and a widened mediastinum on chest x-ray or computed tomographic scan. Pleural effusions are also commonly seen. Treatment involves ciprofloxacin (preferred), 400 mg IV every 12 hours, or doxycycline, 100 mg IV every 12 hours, plus one or two additional antibiotics: one antibiotic with good central nervous system penetration, such as rifampin, ampicillin, or meropenem; and clindamycin (due to its potential inhibition of toxin production). Cutaneous anthrax presents with a black scab or eschar surrounded by edema and erythema. It is usually not tender. The treatment reflects the less serious nature of the infection: oral ciprofloxacin, 500 mg twice daily, or doxycycline, 100 mg twice daily. Options for postexposure prophylaxis include oral ciprofloxacin, 500 mg twice daily, or doxycycline, 100 mg twice daily for 60 days. Anthrax is not spread from person to person; only those exposed to the spores from a release site are at risk for infection.[19]

Plague: The classic case presents with fever and chills, followed by an intense swelling and tenderness of the lymph nodes (bubo) in one area (inguinal,

TABLE 7-2 Radionuclide Chelating Agents

Radionuclide	Agent	Dose	Timing of First Dose*
Plutonium, transuranics	Pentetic acid or diethylene triamine pentaacetic acid (DTPA)	1 g IV; may also be inhaled; may be needed daily for weeks	Within 6 h
Cesium, thallium	Prussian blue	1 g orally 3 times daily; may be needed for months	Within 6 h; timing less critical
Uranium	Bicarbonate Potassium chloride	4 g, then 2 g every 4 h until urine pH 8–9	Within 4 h; timing less critical
Iodine 131	Potassium iodide	Adult, 130 mg tablet; age 3–18 y, 65 mg; age 1 month–3 y, 32 mg; age < 1 mo, 16 mg	Within 4 h

* To be most effective.

axillary, or cervical regions). However, in a bioterrorist attack with aerosol spray, pneumonic plague would be the most likely outcome, with fever, cough, and a rapidly progressive pneumonia. The treatment for plague is streptomycin, 1 g IM every 12 hours for 10 days, or doxycycline, 100 mg twice daily (IV or orally) for 7 to 10 days. The postexposure prophylaxis is doxycycline, 100 mg orally twice daily for 7 days. Plague is spread by droplets, so anyone within 3 feet of an infected person is at risk of developing the disease, as is anyone exposed at the release site.[20]

Tularemia: The classic case presents with fever and a tender papule (raised bump). The papule develops an ulcerated center with an eschar (scab), and tender lymph nodes emerge in the area of drainage of the skin lesion. In a bioterrorist attack with aerosol spray, tularemia may present as the sudden development of sepsis with fever and shock, with or without a rapidly progressive pneumonia, and without the classic skin lesions and lymphadenopathy. Though the treatment for an individual patient is streptomycin, 1 g IM twice daily for 10 days, or gentamicin, 5 mg/kg, mass casualty treatment or postexposure prophylaxis uses doxycycline, 100 mg orally twice daily, or ciprofloxacin, 500 mg orally twice daily for 14 days. Tularemia is not spread from person to person, so only those exposed to the bacteria from a release site are at risk.[21]

Smallpox: Smallpox presents with a fever and rash that starts as macules (raised, flat, broad, erythematous bumps) and evolves into pustules, initially appearing on the face and extremities, including the palms and soles, and spreading to the trunk. All lesions are at the same stage of development (as opposed to chickenpox, in which the lesions are at different stages) and the pustules tend to be rounded, 5 mm in diameter, and umbilicated. Treatment is only supportive care. The smallpox vaccine is effective prophylaxis if given within 72 hours after exposure (see Appendix). Smallpox is an airborne virus and is spread easily from person to person by air or contact.[22]

Viral hemorrhagic fever: These viruses present with fever, "red eyes" due to conjunctival hemorrhage, a maculopapular rash, and melena. Care is supportive. Oral ribavirin may be used in mass casualty situations, though it may be useful for only two of the four families of viral hemorrhagic fever (arenaviruses and bunyaviruses). There is also no known effective postexposure prophylaxis. These viruses are highly contagious via contact. Although airborne spread has not been demonstrated, this possibility has not been conclusively excluded.[23]

Botulism: Botulism presents as a descending paralysis that starts in the facial area and moves caudally. Botulism antitoxin will stop the progression of paralysis but will not reverse existing paralysis. If the respiratory muscles have been involved, then ventilatory support will be required until the effects of the botulinum toxin have resolved, which may take 1 to 3 months. Botulism is secondary to the toxin and not the bacteria itself, so there is no person-to-person spread of botulism.[20]

As shown in Table 7-3, most class A biologic agents present with fever. As opposed to most chemical casualties, biologic casualties usually have delayed onset of respiratory symptoms.[24] Mass biologic casualties will significantly overwhelm antibiotic and critical care resources.

TABLE 7-3 Differentiation of Category A Biologic Casualties

Symptoms & signs	Anthrax	Plague	Tularemia	Smallpox	Viral Hemorrhagic Fever	Botulism
Fever	XX	XX	XX	XX	XX	
Chest discomfort	XX					
Cough	XX + blood	XX	XX + blood		X + blood	
Bubos		XX				
Myalgias				XX	XX	
Pustules				Same stage		
Hemorrhage					XX	
Descending paralysis						XX

X's indicate degree of symptom/sign expression.

7.11 SUMMARY

In the darkest hours of the ill-fated Apollo 13 mission, Gene Krantz asserted, "Failure is not an option." This thinking reflects the quintessential disaster mindset that adapts to adverse situations and overcomes obstacles. Effective mass casualty management begins with an understanding of ideal individual casualty management and moves to application of this knowledge in the context of lethal mechanisms of disaster, high-risk environments for health care responders, limited resources, and a sizeable casualty population. Reaching the greatest good for the casualty population then becomes achievable.

REFERENCES

1. Chambers J, Purdue G. Radiation injury and the surgeon. *J Am Coll Surg.* 2007;204(1); 128–139.

2. Daugherty E. Health care worker protection in mass casualty respiratory failure: infection control, decontamination, and personal protective equipment. *Respir Care.* 2008;53(2): 201–212.

3. Centers for Disease Control and Prevention. Radiological Terrorism, Emergency Management Pocket Guide for Clinicians. 2005. www.bt.cdc.gov/radiation/pocket.asp. Accessed November 27, 2010.

4. Mettler F, Voelz G, Major radiation exposure—what to expect and how to respond. *N Engl J Med.* 2002;346(20);1554–1561.

5. Kales S, Christiani D. Acute chemical emergencies. *N Engl J Med.* 2004;350(8);800–808.

6. Tur-Kaspa I, Lev E, Hendler I, et al. Preparing hospitals for toxicological mass casualties events. *Crit Care Med.* 1999;27(5):1004–1008.

7. DePalma R, Burris D, Champion H, Hodgson M. Blast injuries. *N Engl J Med.* 2005;352(13):1335–1342.

8. Wightman J, Gladish S. Explosions and blast injuries. *Ann Emerg Med.* 2001;37(6):664–678.

9. Blast injuries: ear blast injuries. http://www.bt.cdc.gov/masscasualties/blastinjury-ear.asp. Accessed September 12, 2010.

10. Ritenour A, Wickley A, Ritenour J, et al. Tympanic membrane perforation and hearing loss from blast overpressure in Operation Enduring Freedom and Operation Iraqi Freedom wounded. *J Trauma.* 2008; 64(2):S174–S178.

11. Welling D, Burris D, Hutton J, Minken S, Rich N. A balanced approach to tourniquet use; lessons learned and relearned. *J Am Coll Surg.* 2006;203(1):106–115.

12. Blast injuries: crush injuries and crush syndrome. http://www.bt.cdc.gov/masscasualties/ blastinjury-crush.asp. Accessed November 1, 2009.

13. Sever M, Vanholder R, Lameire N. Management of crush-related injuries after disaster. *N Engl J Med.* 2006;354:1052–1063.

14. Richards C, Wallis D. Asphyxiation: a review. *Trauma.* 2005;7:37–45.

15. Barillo D, Wolf S. Planning for burn disasters: lessons learned from one hundred years of history. *J Burn Care Res.* 2006;27(5):622–634.

16. Multiservice Tactics, Techniques, and Procedures for Treatment of Chemical Agent Casualties and Conventional Military Chemical Injuries, FM 8–285. September 2007. http://www.fas.org/irp/doddir/army/fm4-02-285.pdf. Accessed August 2, 2010.

17. *Medical Management of Chemical Casualties.* 3rd ed. Aberdeen Proving Ground, MD: US Army Medical Research Institute of Chemical Defense; 2000.

18. Medical Treatment of Radiological Casualties. Dept of Homeland Security Working Group on Radiological Dispersal Device Preparedness. http://www.bt.cdc.gov/radiation/clinicians.asp. Accessed October 24, 2009.

19. Inglesby T, O'Toole T, Henderson D, et al. Anthrax as a biological weapon, 2002: updated recommendations for Management. *JAMA.* 2002;287:2236–2252.

20. Fry D, Schecter W, Parker J, et al. The surgeon and acts of civilian terrorism: biologic agents. *J Am Coll Surg.* 2005;200(2):291–302.

21. Dennis D, Inglesby T, Henderson D, et al. Tularemia as a biological weapon: medical and public health management. *JAMA.* 2001;285:2763–2773.

22. Henderson D, Inglesby T, Bartlett J, et al. Smallpox as a biological weapon: medical and public health management. *JAMA.* 1999;281:2127–2137.

23. Borio L, Inglesby T, Peters C, et al. Hemorrhagic fever viruses as biological weapons: medical and public health management. *JAMA.* 2002;287:2391–2405.

24. Cieslak T, Rowe J, Kortepeter M, et al. A field-expedient algorithmic approach to the clinical management of chemical and biological casualties. *Milit Med.* 2000;165:659–622.

25. *Advanced Trauma Life Support.* 8th ed. Chicago, IL: American College of Surgeons; 2008.

26. Armstrong J, Ziglar M. Florida Standardized Tourniquet Protocol. http://www.faemsmd.org/ pdfs/DRAFTStandardizedTourniquetProtocol.pdf. Accessed December 15, 2009.

27. Smallpox Vaccination and Adverse Events Training Module. www.bt.cdc.gov/training/ smallpoxvaccine/reactions. Accessed August 2, 2010.

28. http://www.duodote.com/index.asp. Accessed April 19, 2011.

APPENDIX. MASS CASUALTY MANAGEMENT SKILLS

A. Needle chest decompression[25]

1. Indication: tension pneumothorax

2. Diagnosis: pneumothorax (absent breath sounds) + hypotension

3. Performance

   ➤ Identify the second intercostal space, midclavicular line on the affected side (Figure 7-3).

   ➤ When possible, conduct quick skin preparation.

   ➤ Insert a 7-cm 12- to 14-gauge over-the-needle catheter over the rib in the second intercostal space, midclavicular line, and into the pleural space on the affected hemithorax.

   ➤ A gush of air and improvement in vital signs (blood pressure, pulse) confirms the diagnosis of tension pneumothorax.

   ➤ Remove the needle and leave the catheter in place.

   ➤ Stabilize the catheter on the chest wall.

   ➤ This procedure converts an emergency into an urgency for subsequent chest tube placement.

FIGURE 7-3
Right needle chest decompression

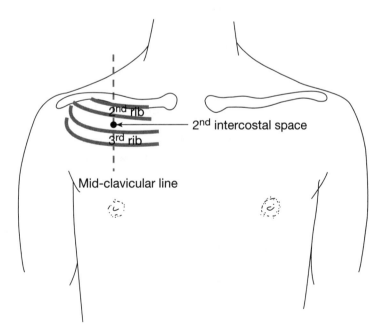

Courtesy of Jodie A. Armstrong, MD.

B. Tourniquet placement[26]

1. Indications for tourniquet use: to stop bleeding when

   ➤ Life-threatening limb hemorrhage is not controlled with direct pressure or other simple measures, as may occur with a mangled extremity.

   ➤ Traumatic amputation has occurred.

2. Application of the combat application tourniquet (CAT)

   ➤ Expose the extremity by removing clothing in proximity to the injury.

   ➤ Place tourniquet directly over exposed skin at least 5 cm proximal to the injury.

   ➤ Route the self-adhering band around the extremity.

   ➤ Pass the band through the outside slit of the buckle.

   ➤ Pull the self-adhering band tight.

   ➤ Twist the rod until bright red bleeding stops.

   ➤ Lock the rod in place with the clip.

   ➤ Record the date and time of application on the tourniquet.

3. Evaluation of effective application

   ➤ Cessation of bleeding from the injured extremity, indicating total occlusion of arterial blood flow.

   ➤ Absence of any preexisting distal pulse.

4. Tourniquet time and removal

   ➤ Tourniquets should be removed as soon as possible under conditions where the hemorrhage can be directly controlled.

   ➤ Tourniquet placement must be communicated in patient reports for all prehospital to hospital and interhospital transfers.

   ➤ Tourniquet time greater than 6 hours is associated with distal tissue loss.

5. Training: Appropriate tourniquet use requires initial and annual renewal training *with skill demonstration.*

6. Outcomes: Tourniquet use should be tracked via institutional and state-wide reporting registries. The indication, specific tourniquet used, time in place, limb injury, mortality, limb loss, and tourniquet-related complications should be included.

C. Administration of nerve agent antidote kit (DuoDote, Mark I)[16]

1. The DuoDote kit consists of a single auto-injector cartridge that contains both 2 mg of atropine and 600 mg of pralidoxime chloride (2-PAM). The Mark I kit contains two auto-injector cartridges; the smaller one has 2 mg of atropine and the larger one has 600 mg of pralidoxime chloride (2-PAM). These are held together by a plastic clip.

2. Indication: symptomatic nerve agent exposure

3. Steps

   ➤ Check site: outer thigh muscle, away from hip and knee joints. In thin individuals, the upper outer buttock should be the site.

   ➤ DuoDote[28]

      i. Hold DuoDote in dominant hand with green tip down.

      ii. Pull off gray safety release with non-dominant hand.

      iii. Firmly push the green tip (needle end) at a 90° angle into outer mid-thigh.

      iv. Remove DuoDote and verify injection by visualizing the needle. If needle is not visible, ensure that gray safety release has been removed and repeat injection.

   ➤ Mark 1

      i. Hold Mark-1 with nondominant hand (Figure 7-4).

      ii. Remove small injector (atropine) from clip.

      iii. Inject atropine at injection site by applying even pressure to the injector; do not jab the site. Hold in place for 10 seconds.

      iv. Remove large injector (2-PAM) from clip.

      v. Inject 2-PAM at injection site by applying even pressure to the injector; do not jab the site. Hold in place for 10 seconds.

      vi. Massage injection site.

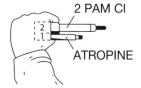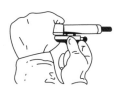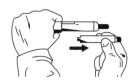

FIGURE 7-4
Mark I Auto-injector Grasp

➤ Attach, if possible, the used cartridges to casualty clothing.

➤ Assess for response; repeat if symptoms still present in 15 minutes. Titrate to breathing and reduction of secretions.

D. Smallpox vaccination[27]

1. Vaccinia (smallpox) vaccine is a live virus that does not contain variola, the virus that causes smallpox.

2. Vaccination

➤ Use no alcohol or other skin preparation.

➤ Dip sterile bifurcated needle into vaccine vial.

➤ Make 15 perpendicular, vigorous insertions within a 5-mm diameter area over the deltoid of the upper arm.

➤ Absorb excess with gauze.

➤ Cover site with sterile gauze.

➤ Discard all materials as infectious waste.

➤ Prevent contact transmission—the virus propagates in the skin and thus is a contamination risk.

3. Normal reaction timeline (a "take")

➤ Day 3–4   Papule

➤ Day 5–6   Vesicle with erythema

➤ Day 8–9   Discrete pustule

➤ Day 12+   Scab

➤ Day 17–21   Scab detaches

4. Normal variants

➤ Satellite lesions

➤ Lymphangitis and regional lymphadenopathy

➤ Marked local site edema

➤ Intense site erythema

5. *No* reaction indicates *no* immunity; vaccination should be repeated.

Appendices

PRE-DISASTER Paradigm™ and DISASTER Paradigm™

PRE-DISASTER Paradigm™

P	Planning and Practice	Do your community and workplace have disaster plans? Do you have a personal or family plan? Are these plans practiced and updated regularly?
R	Resilience	What measures are in place to help individuals, organizations, and communities cope with the environmental and psychological consequences of disaster?
E	Education	What can you do to prepare for disaster through competency-based, inter-professional education and training in disaster medicine and public health preparedness?

DISASTER Paradigm™

D	Detect	Do needs exceed resources? Who is notified that a disaster is happening?
I	Incident Management	What is your role? Who is the incident commander?
S	Scene Safety/Security	Is the scene secure? Is it safe to enter?
A	Assess Hazards	Fire? Hazardous materials? Radiation? Building collapse? Downed power lines? Secondary devices? Contaminated casualties?
S	Support	What outside assistance is needed (eg, police, fire, emergency medical services, government, other)? Can adequate surge capability and capacity be established to meet local public safety/health needs and priorities?
T	Triage and Treatment	Are protocols, procedures, and resources in place for the rapid triage and immediate treatment of casualties? What public health interventions are needed?
E	Evacuation	Are enough transport units en route to the scene? Should affected people evacuate or shelter-in-place?
R	Recovery	Has critical infrastructure been damaged? What are the short- and long-term health needs of casualties and affected populations?

Competencies for Health Professionals in Disaster Medicine and Public Health Preparedness, with Specific Reference to ADLS

Source: Subbarao I, Lyznicki J, Hsu E, et al. A Consensus-based Educational Framework and Competency Set for the Discipline of Disaster Medicine and Public Health Preparedness. 2008; 2:57–68.

Competency Domains	Core Competencies	Category-Specific Competencies		
		Informed Worker/Student	Practitioner	Leader
1.0 Preparation and Planning	1.1 Demonstrate proficiency in the use of an all-hazards framework for disaster planning and mitigation.	1.1.1 Describe the all-hazards framework for disaster planning and mitigation. 1.1.2 Explain key components of regional, community, institutional, and personal/family disaster plans.	1.1.3 Summarize your regional, community, office, institutional, and personal/family disaster plans. 1.1.4 Explain the purpose of disaster exercises and drills in regional, community, and institutional disaster preparation and planning. 1.1.5 Conduct hazard vulnerability assessments for your office practice, community, or institution.	1.1.6 Participate in the design, implementation, and evaluation of regional, community, and institutional disaster plans.
	1.2 Demonstrate proficiency in addressing the health-related needs, values, and perspectives of all ages and populations in regional, community, and institutional disaster plans.	1.2.1 Identify individuals (of all ages) and populations with special needs who may be more vulnerable to adverse health effects in a disaster or public health emergency.	1.2.2 Delineate health care and public health issues that need to be addressed in regional, community, and institutional disaster plans to accommodate the needs, values, and perspectives of all ages and populations. 1.2.3 Identify psychological reactions that may be exhibited by victims of all ages, their families, and responders in a disaster or public health emergency.	1.2.4 Create, evaluate, and revise policies and procedures for meeting the health-related needs of all ages and populations in regional, community, and institutional disaster plans.

2.0 Detection and Communication	2.1 Demonstrate proficiency in the detection of and immediate response to a disaster or public health emergency.	2.1.1 Recognize general indicators and epidemiologic clues of a disaster or public health emergency (including natural, unintentional, and terrorist events). 2.1.2 Describe immediate actions and precautions to protect yourself and others from harm in a disaster or public health emergency.	2.1.3 Characterize signs and symptoms, as well as disease and injury patterns, likely to be associated with exposure to natural disasters or to conventional and nuclear explosives and/or release of biologic, chemical, and radiologic agents. 2.1.4 Explain the purpose and role of surveillance systems that can be used to detect and monitor a disaster or public health emergency.	2.1.5 Evaluate and modify policies and procedures for the detection and immediate response to natural disasters, industrial- or transportation-related catastrophes (eg, hazardous material spill, explosion), epidemics, and acts of terrorism (eg, involving conventional and nuclear explosives and/or release of biologic, chemical, and radiologic agents).
	2.2 Demonstrate proficiency in the use of information and communication systems in a disaster or public health emergency.	2.2.1 Describe emergency communication and reporting systems and procedures for contacting family members, relatives, coworkers, and local authorities in a disaster or public health emergency. 2.2.2 Describe informational resources that are available for health professionals and the public to prepare for, respond to, and recover from disasters.	2.2.3 Utilize emergency communications systems to report critical health information to appropriate authorities in a disaster or public health emergency. 2.2.4 Access timely and credible health and safety information for all ages and populations affected by natural disasters, industrial- or transportation-related catastrophes (eg, hazardous material spill, explosion), epidemics, and acts of terrorism (eg, involving conventional and nuclear explosives and/or release of biologic, chemical, and radiologic agents).	2.2.5 Evaluate and modify risk communication and emergency reporting systems to ensure that health, safety, and security warnings and actions taken are articulated clearly and appropriately in a disaster or public health emergency.

(continued)

2.3 Demonstrate proficiency in addressing cultural, ethnic, religious, linguistic, socioeconomic, and special health-related needs of all ages and populations in regional, community, and institutional emergency communication systems.

2.3.1 Describe strategies for and barriers to communicating and disseminating health information to all ages and populations affected by a disaster or public health emergency.

2.3.2 Delineate cultural, ethnic, religious, linguistic, and health-related issues that need to be addressed in regional, community, and institutional emergency communication systems for all ages and populations affected by a disaster or public health emergency.

2.3.3 Create, evaluate, and revise policies and procedures for meeting the needs of all ages and populations in regional, community, and institutional emergency communication systems.

3.0 Incident Management and Support Systems

3.1 Demonstrate proficiency in the initiation, deployment, and coordination of national, regional, state, local, and institutional incident command and emergency operations systems.

3.1.1 Describe the purpose and relevance of the National Response Plan, National Incident Management System, and Hospital Incident Command System, and Emergency Support Function-8 to regional, community, and institutional disaster response.

3.1.2 Delineate your function and describe other job functions in institutional, community, and regional disaster response systems to ensure unified command and scalable response to a disaster or public health emergency.

3.1.3 Perform your expected role in a disaster (eg, through participation in exercises and drills) within the incident or emergency management system established by the community, organization, or institution.

3.1.4 Devise, evaluate, and modify institutional, community, and regional incident command, emergency operations, and emergency response systems (eg, based on after-action reports from actual events, disaster exercises, and drills) to ensure unified command and scalable response to a disaster or public health emergency.

3.2 Demonstrate proficiency in the mobilization and coordination of disaster support services.	3.2.1 Describe global, federal, regional, state, local, institutional, organizational, and private industry disaster support services, including the rationale for the integration and coordination of these systems.	3.2.2 Demonstrate the ability to collaborate with relevant public and private sector stakeholders to ensure efficient coordination of civilian, military, and other disaster response assets.	3.2.3 Develop, evaluate, and revise policies and procedures for mobilizing and integrating global, federal, regional, state, local, institutional, organizational, and private industry disaster support services in a disaster. This includes knowledge of legal statutes and mutual aid agreements for the mobilization and deployment of civilian, military, and other response personnel and assets.
3.3 Demonstrate proficiency in the provision of health system surge capacity for the management of mass casualties in a disaster or public health emergency.	3.3.1 Describe the potential impact of mass casualties on access to and availability of clinical and public health resources in a disaster.	3.3.2 Characterize institutional, community, and regional surge capacity assets in the public and private health response sectors and the extent of their potential assistance in a disaster or public health emergency.	3.3.3 Develop and evaluate policies, plans, and strategies for predicting and providing surge capacity of institutional, community, and regional health systems for the management of mass casualties in a disaster or public health emergency.

(continued)

4.0 Safety and Security	4.1 Demonstrate proficiency in the prevention and mitigation of health, safety, and security risks to yourself and others in a disaster.	4.1.1 Using an all-hazards framework, explain general health, safety, and security risks associated with disasters.	4.1.2 Characterize unique health, safety, and security risks associated with natural disasters, industrial- or transportation-related catastrophes (eg, hazardous material spill, explosion), epidemics, and acts of terrorism (eg, involving conventional and nuclear explosives and/or release of biologic chemical, and radiologic agents).	4.1.3 Develop, evaluate, and revise community, institutional, and regional policies and procedures to protect the health, safety, and security of all ages and populations affected by a disaster or public health emergency.
		4.1.2 Describe infection control precautions to protect health care workers, other responders, and the public from exposure to communicable diseases, such as pandemic influenza.	4.1.3 Utilize federal and institutional guidelines and protocols to prevent the transmission of infectious agents in health care and community settings.	
	4.2 Demonstrate proficiency in the selection and use of personal protective equipment at a disaster scene or receiving facility.	4.2.1 Describe the rationale, function, and limitations of personal protective equipment that may be used in a disaster or public health emergency.	4.2.2 Demonstrate the ability to select, locate, don, and work in personal protective equipment according to the degree and type of protection required for various types of exposures.	4.2.3 Develop, evaluate, and revise policies, protocols, and procedures for the use of all levels of personal protective equipment that may be used at a disaster scene or receiving facility.
	4.3 Demonstrate proficiency in victim decontamination at a disaster scene or receiving facility.	4.3.1 Explain the purpose of victim decontamination in a disaster.	4.3.2 Decontaminate victims at a disaster scene or receiving facility.	4.3.3 Develop, evaluate, and revise decontamination policies, protocols, and procedures that may be implemented at a disaster scene or receiving facility.

5.0 Clinical/ Public Health Assessment and Intervention	5.1 Demonstrate proficiency in the use of triage systems in a disaster or public health emergency.	5.1.1 Explain the role of triage as a basis for prioritizing or rationing health care services for victims and communities affected by a disaster or public health emergency.	5.1.2 Explain the strengths and limitations of various triage systems that have been developed for the management of mass casualties at a disaster scene or receiving facility. 5.1.3 Perform mass casualty triage at a disaster scene or receiving facility.	5.1.5 Develop, evaluate, and revise mass casualty and population-based triage policies, protocols, and procedures that may be implemented in a disaster or public health emergency.
	5.2 Demonstrate proficiency in the clinical assessment and management of injuries, illnesses, and mental health conditions manifested by all ages and populations in a disaster or public health emergency.	5.2.1 Describe possible medical and mental health consequences for all ages and populations affected by a disaster or public health emergency. 5.2.2 Explain basic lifesaving and support principles and procedures that can be utilized at a disaster scene.	5.2.3 Demonstrate the ability to apply and adapt clinical knowledge and skills for the assessment and management of injuries and illnesses in victims of all ages under various exposure scenarios (eg, natural disasters; industrial- or transportation-related catastrophes; epidemics; and acts of terrorism involving conventional and nuclear explosives and/or release of biologic, chemical, and radiologic agents), in accordance with professional scope of practice. 5.2.4 Identify strategies to manage fear, panic, stress, and other psychological responses that may be elicited by victims, families, and responders in a disaster or public health emergency.	5.2.5 Develop, evaluate, and revise policies, protocols, and procedures for the clinical care of all ages and populations under crisis conditions, with limited situational awareness and resources.

(continued)

5.3 Demonstrate proficiency in the management of mass fatalities in a disaster or public health emergency.

5.3.1 Describe psychological, emotional, cultural, religious, and forensic considerations for the management of mass fatalities in a disaster or public health emergency.

5.3.2 Explain the implications of and specialized support services required for the management of mass fatalities from natural disasters, epidemics, and acts of terrorism (eg, involving conventional and nuclear explosives and/or release of biologic, chemical, and radiologic agents).

5.3.3 Explain the significance of (and the need to collect and preserve) forensic evidence from living and deceased humans and animals at a disaster scene or receiving facility.

5.3.4 Develop, evaluate, and revise policies, protocols, and procedures for the management of human and animal remains at a disaster scene or receiving facility.

5.4 Demonstrate proficiency in public health interventions to protect the health of all ages, populations, and communities affected by a disaster or public health emergency.

5.4.1 Describe short- and long-term public health interventions appropriate for all ages, populations, and communities affected by a disaster or public health emergency.

5.4.2 Apply knowledge and skills for the public health management of all ages, populations, and communities affected by natural disasters, industrial- or transportation-related catastrophes, epidemics, and acts of terrorism, in accordance with professional scope of practice. This includes active and passive surveillance, movement restriction, vector control, mass immunization and prophylaxis, rapid needs assessment, environmental monitoring, safety of food and water, and sanitation.

5.4.3 Develop, evaluate, and revise public health policies, protocols, and procedures for the management of all ages, populations, and communities affected by natural disasters, industrial- or transportation-related catastrophes, epidemics, and acts of terrorism.

6.0 Contingency, Continuity, and Recovery	6.1 Demonstrate proficiency in the application of contingency interventions for all ages, populations, institutions, and communities affected by a disaster or public health emergency.	6.1.1 Describe solutions for ensuring the continuity of supplies and services to meet your medical and mental health needs, as well as those of your family, office practice, institution, and community in a disaster, under various contingency situations (eg, mass evacuation, mass sheltering, prolonged shelter-in-place).	6.1.2 Demonstrate creative and flexible decision making in various contingency situations and risk scenarios, under crisis conditions and with limited situational awareness.	6.1.4 Develop, evaluate, and revise contingency and continuity policies and plans for health professionals, institutions, and community health systems to maintain the highest possible standards of care under various risk scenarios.
			6.1.3 Describe community and institutional protocols and procedures for the evacuation and transport of individuals and populations (of all ages) affected by a disaster or public health emergency.	
	6.2 Demonstrate proficiency in the application of recovery solutions for all ages, populations, institutions, and communities affected by a disaster or public health emergency.	6.2.1 Describe short- and long-term medical and mental health considerations for the recovery of all ages, populations, and communities affected by a disaster or public health emergency.	6.2.2 Describe solutions for ensuring the recovery of clinical records, supplies, and services to meet your physical and mental health needs, as well as those of your family, institution, and community in a disaster or public health emergency.	6.2.4 Develop, evaluate, and revise policies, plans, and procedures for the continual evaluation of regional, community, and institutional disaster response and recovery efforts, and implement necessary actions to enhance health system preparedness, response, and recovery for future events.
			6.2.3 Explain mechanisms for providing postevent feedback and lessons learned to appropriate authorities (eg, through after-action reports) to improve regional, community, and institutional disaster response systems.	

(continued)

| 7.0 Public Health Law and Ethics | 7.1 Demonstrate proficiency in the application of moral and ethical principles and policies for ensuring access to and availability of health services for all ages, populations, and communities affected by a disaster or public health emergency. | 7.1.1 Describe moral and ethical issues relevant to the management of individuals (of all ages), populations, and communities affected by a disaster or public health emergency. | 7.1.2 Apply moral and ethical principles and policies to address individual and community health needs in a disaster. This includes understanding of professional obligation to treat, the right to protect personal safety in a disaster, and responsibilities and rights of health professionals in a disaster or public health emergency. | 7.1.3 Develop, evaluate, and revise ethical principles, policies, and codes to address individual and community health needs in all disaster phases. |
| | 7.2 Demonstrate proficiency in the application of laws and regulations to protect the health and safety of all ages, populations, and communities affected by a disaster or public health emergency. | 7.2.1 Describe legal and regulatory issues relevant to disasters and public health emergencies, including the basic legal framework for public health. | 7.2.2 Apply legal principles, policies, and practices to address individual and community health needs in a disaster. This includes understanding of liability, worker protection and compensation, licensure, privacy, quarantine laws, and other legal issues to enable and encourage health professionals to participate in disaster response and maintain the highest possible standards of care under extreme conditions. | 7.2.3 Develop, evaluate, and revise legal principles, policies, practices, and codes to address individual and community health needs in all disaster phases. |

List of Acronyms and Abbreviations

LIST OF ACRONYMS AND ABBREVIATIONS

AAR	After action report
ACF	Alternate care facility
ADLS	Advanced Disaster Life Support
ATSDR	Agency for Toxic Substances and Disease Registry
BAL	British anti-lewisite [agent]
BSL	Biosafety level
CDC	Centers for Disease Control and Prevention
CERT	Community Emergency Response Team
COCA	Clinician Outreach and Communication Activity
DDD	Defined daily doses
DHHS	Department of Health and Human Services
DHS	Department of Homeland Security
DISASTER paradigm	Detect; Incident command; Scene security and safety; Assess hazards; Support; Triage and treatment; Evacuation; Recovery
DMAT	Disaster medical assistance team
DMORT	Disaster mortuary operational response team
DTAC	Disaster Technical Assistance Center
EM	Emergency management
EMAC	Emergency Management Assistance Compact
EMS	Emergency medical services
EMTALA	Emergency Medical Treatment and Active Labor Act
EOC	Emergency Operations Center
ESAR-VHP	Emergency System for Advance Registration of Volunteer Health Professionals
ESF	Emergency support function
FAC	Family Assistance Center
FBI	Federal Bureau of Investigation
FEMA	Federal Emergency Management Agency
HAMR	Health and Medical Response
HAN	Health Alert Network
HAZMAT	Hazardous materials
HEOC	Health Emergency Operations Center
HEPA	High-efficiency particulate air
HHS	US Department of Health and Human Services

HICS	Hospital Incident Command System
HRSA	Health Resources and Services Administration
HSPD	Homeland Security Presidential Directive
IC	Incident command
IDLH	Immediately dangerous to life and health
IOM	Institute of Medicine
IP	Improvement plan
JIC	Joint information center
LRN	Laboratory Response Network
MCE	Mass casualty event
MCI	Mass casualty incident
MSDS	Material safety data sheet
MEC	Medical examiner/coroner
MQS	Minimum qualifications of survival
MRC	Medical Reserve Corps
MSCC	Medical Surge Capacity and Capability [Management System]
NDLS	National Disaster Life Support
NDMS	National Disaster Medical System
NFMC	National Foundation of Mortuary Care
NIMS	National Incident Management System
NIOSH	National Institutes for Occupational Safety and Health
NRF	National Response Framework
NTSB	National Transportation Safety Board
OAFME	Office of Armed Forces Medical Examiner
OSHA	Occupational Health and Safety Administration
PALS	Prevention, Access, Life Support, and Specialized Care
PAPR	Powered air purifying respirator
PBI	Pulmonary blast injury
PEL	Permissible exposure limit
PHSCC	Public Health Services Commission Corps
PICE	Potential injury- and/or illness-creating events
PPE	Personal protective equipment
PRE-DISASTER	Planning and practice, resilience, and education and training DISASTER [paradigm]
RDF	Rapid Deployment Force
RNA	Rapid needs assessment

RT-PCR	Reverse transcriptase polymerase chain reaction
SALT	Sort, assess, life-saving interventions, and treatment/transport
SAMHSA	Substance Abuse and Mental Health Services Administration
SARS	Severe acute respiratory syndrome
SAVE	Secondary Assessment of Victim Endpoint
SEIRV	*S*usceptible, *e*xposed, *i*nfectious, *r*emoved by death or illness recovery, or *v*accine protected
SNS	Strategic National Stockpile
SOFA	Sequential Organ Failure Assessment
TJC	The Joint Commission
UEVHPA	Uniform Emergency Volunteer Health Professionals Act
WHO	World Health Organization

ADLS GLOSSARY

All-hazards preparedness: Planning that considers all potential hazards to a community and that moves a community to mitigate against, and practice response for, any potential hazard that may affect the community

Alternative care sites: Facilities that can be used in a disaster to care for "overflow" patients transferred from large hospitals and trauma centers to make room for more acutely injured casualties

Biosafety level (BSL) classification: System used to determine the types of agents scientists can work with, the extent of testing they can perform, and the safety precautions that must be in place to protect workers and prevent the release of potentially dangerous microorganisms into the environment

Capacity assessment: Identifying available resources that can be used to reduce risk, enhance survival, and help casualties and populations cope with disasters

Combined disaster: A catastrophic event characterized by a combination of natural, technological, and/or conflict-based disasters

Conflict-based disaster: A disaster resulting from the intentional creation of human insecurity by actual or threatened terrorism, civil disorder along political, ethnic, religious, or economic lines, or war with large-scale loss of life

Containment: The process of defining and containing an infectious disease outbreak in specific geographic regions so as to isolate individuals and communities that are infected with the virus and prevent further transmission, in accordance with a plan developed by the World Health Organization

Contingency capacity: Spaces, staff, and supplies not used in daily practice, yet functionally equivalent to usual practice, that may be used temporarily during a major mass casualty incident and on a more sustained basis during a disaster

Conventional capacity: Spaces, staff, and supplies used in daily practice within an institution

Crisis capacity: Adaptive spaces, staff, and supplies outside usual standards of care, yet sufficient (ie, the best possible care to casualties given the circumstances and resources available) in the setting of a catastrophic disaster

Crush syndrome: Localized crush injury with systemic manifestations

Disaster: A serious disruption of the functioning of society, causing widespread human, material, or environmental losses that exceed the ability of affected society to cope by using only its own resources (World Association of Disaster and Emergency Medicine); an occurrence of a natural catastrophe, technological accident, or human-caused event that has resulted in severe property damage, deaths, and/or multiple injuries (FEMA); an event and its consequences that results in a serious disruption of the functioning of a community and causing widespread human, material, economic, or environmental losses that exceed the capacity of the affected area to respond without external assistance to save lives, preserve property, and maintain the stability and integrity of the affected area (NDLS Education Consortium)

Dirty bomb: A non-nuclear explosive combined with radioactive material to create local injury and induce widespread panic

DISASTER Paradigm™: A mnemonic that organizes interprofessional providers' planning for and response to a disaster: D, detect; I, incident management; S, security and safety; A, assess hazards; S, support; T, triage and treatment; E, evacuation; R, recovery

Disaster taxonomy: Classification of disasters based on distinguishing characteristics and common relationships across hazards

Dry decontamination: The act of removing garments that are superficially contaminated or have retained vapor within them

Epidemic: A situation with more cases of a disease than usual in a defined geographic area

ESF-6: Emergency support function for mass care, emergency assistance, housing, and human services

ESF-8: Emergency support function for public health and medical services

Expectant casualties: Disaster casualties who are still alive, but are so severely injured they have little chance of survival either absolutely (eg, 100% body surface area burns) or relatively given the available resources

Extremity compartment syndrome: A syndrome resulting from increased pressure within the fascial compartments of an extremity, leading to neurovascular and organ compromise

Heat cramps: Muscle cramps in the extremities and trunk due to electrolyte imbalance

Heat exhaustion: A condition marked by fatigue, nausea, and fainting, due to dehydration associated with ambient temperature elevation

Heat stroke: A medical emergency that occurs when the body's system of temperature regulation fails and body temperature rises to critical levels

Incident management: The way in which incidents are managed across all Homeland Security activities, including prevention, protection, response, mitigation, and recovery

Isolation: Placement of people known to have a communicable disease in a separate area where they will not expose others

Mass care: The coordination of nonmedical services to include sheltering of displaced persons, organizing feeding operations, providing emergency first aid at designated sites, collecting and providing information on casualties to family members, and coordinating bulk distribution of emergency relief items

Mass casualty event: The direct medical consequence of a disaster, in which the casualty load overwhelms available resources

Mass casualty incident: The direct medical consequence of a disaster in which the casualty load strains, but does not overwhelm, available resources

Mass fatality event: An event that produces fatalities that overwhelm available fatality management resources

Natural disaster: A naturally occurring event or hazard that results in a disaster, such as an earthquake, tornado, or naturally-occurring disease outbreak

Ontario Protocol: A protocol that establishes three criteria through which critical care resource allocation can be determined for each casualty in a prolonged public health emergency: inclusion, exclusion, and minimum qualifications of survival

Over-triage: Assigning non-critically injured casualties to a higher triage category than appropriate, thus applying scarce resources to casualties who do not need them at that time

Pandemic: A global epidemic of a disease

Potential injury- and/or illness-creating event (PICE): An event that may initially appear to be a static, well-controlled local event and yet may quickly become a regional, national, or global disaster

PRE-DISASTER Paradigm™: Steps to take before a disaster occurs: P, planning and practice; R, resilience; E, education

Public health: A complex network of people, systems, and organizations that work together to ensure the conditions necessary to live healthy lives

Public health emergency: An event that adversely impacts the public health system and/or its protective infrastructure (ie, water, sanitation, shelter, food, fuel, and health), resulting in both direct and indirect consequences to the health of a population

Public health surveillance: The systematic, ongoing assessment of the health of a community, which provides a baseline description of a health problem and the ways in which it changes or evolves

Quarantine: Placement of people exposed to a contagious disease, but currently asymptomatic, in a separate area where they will not expose others and can be monitored for the development of the disease

Reproduction (transmissibility) rate: The average number of secondary cases of a communicable disease generated by a typical primary case in a susceptible population; abbreviated as R0

Reverse triage: The process of rapidly identifying patients who can be safely discharged from a hospital to home, an alternate care site, or a skilled nursing facility

SALT triage system: A disaster triage system that instructs providers to *sort* casualties by their ability to follow commands, individually *assess* casualties and apply *lifesaving interventions* rapidly, and assign a *treatment and/or transport* priority

SEIRV: Population-based triage method for infectious illness, which includes the five categories of *s*usceptible, *e*xposed, *i*nfectious, *r*emoved, and *v*accinated

Social distancing: A community imposes limitations on social (face-to-face) interactions to reduce exposure to and transmission of the disease

Surge capability: The number of casualties who can receive specific services given available personnel skills and resources (ie, number of ventilated patients given available ventilators, ventilator-proficient physicians and nurses, respiratory therapists, and monitored settings)

Surge capacity: The ability to accommodate a sudden, unexpected increase in casualty volume that exceeds the usual capacity of the health care system or facility

Technological disaster: An event resulting from a human systems failure, such as poorly designed buildings or flawed equipment, and human errors due to inadequate training, worker distraction, or fatigue

Triage: Prioritization of care based on the severity of illness or injury, ability to survive, and the resources available

Undertriage: Assigning critically injured casualties to a lower triage category than appropriate because the severity of casualty illness or injury is unrecognized, resulting in delayed treatment

Wet decontamination: The process of washing a grossly contaminated or symptomatic casualty from head to toe with soap and tepid water

INDEX

NOTES

NOTES

NOTES

NOTES

NOTES

NOTES

NOTES

NOTES